Botulinum Toxin in Facial Rejuvenation

SECOND EDITION

Botulinum Toxin in Facial Rejuvenation

KATE COLEMAN BSc, PhD, FRCS, FRCOphth
Blackrock Clinic
Dublin, Ireland

ELSEVIER

BOTULINUM TOXIN IN FACIAL REJUVENATION,
SECOND EDITION

ISBN: 978-0-7020-7786-9

Notices

International Standard Book Number: 978-0-7020-7786-9

Content Strategist: Kayla Wolfe
Content Development Manager: Katie DeFrancesco
Content Development Specialist: Caroline Dorey-Stein
Publishing Services Manager: Shereen Jameel
Project Manager: Nadhiya Sekar
Design Direction: Bridget Hoette

Printed in China

Last digit is the print number: 9 8 7 6 5 4 3 2 1

ELSEVIER

1600 John F. Kennedy Blvd.
Ste 1800
Philadelphia, PA 19103-2899

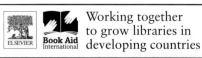

Working together
to grow libraries in
developing countries

www.elsevier.com • www.bookaid.org

FOREWORD, TO THE FIRST EDITION (2003)

It is indeed a great pleasure for us to have the opportunity to write the foreword to this important handbook. Kate Coleman has chronicled and catalogued her extensive observations following the treatment of her patients with botulinum toxin. These are displayed in an orderly fashion, allowing physicians to readily apply these pearls to the treatment of their patients.

We have used botulinum toxin to treat blepharospasm patients for more than 20 years. Now, just as botulinum toxin revolutionised the treatment of benign essential blepharospasm, it is launching noninvasive techniques for facial rejuvenation into another era. Every physician and surgeon seriously pursuing rejuvenation of the facial structures must include chemodenervation as a cornerstone of their therapeutic menu. The effects of ablative and nonablative laser therapies are enhanced with botulinum toxin type A pretreatment. Combination therapy of botulinum toxin and filling agents yields prolonged effacement of glabellar furrows. The artful application of botulinum toxin not only reduces facial rhytidosis but also repositions eyebrows, flattens pretarsal muscle folds and diminishes platysmal bands. Understanding the facial musculature allows the aesthetic physician to manipulate the balance of counteracting muscles and rejuvenate the face. This is the dawn of the new age of facial rejuvenations.

Stephen Bosniak, MD, FACS
New York, NY, USA

Marian Cantisano-Zilkha, MD
Rio de Janeiro, Brazil

Co-editors of *Operative Techniques in Ophthalmic Plastic and Orbital Surgery.*
Authors of *Cosmetic Blepharoplasty and Facial Rejuvenation.*
National Botox Training Centers—New York, NY, USA, and Great Neck, NY, USA.

Thank you to the kind patients who generously donated their photographs and videos, and to the great team at Elsevier for making it happen, again.

Thank you to my mentors whose principles shaped my surgical and clinical problem solving. Professor Leo Koornneef and Dr Stephen Bosniak, may you both be resting in peace enjoying the legacy of new generations of colleagues who now are passing on your teaching.

Little did I think, when I thanked Maria Micheau in the first edition, that she would have remained a rock for all our patients and team, and for me personally. Everyone needs a rock to keep their feet on the ground and their eyes in the heavens; thank you Maria.

Special thanks go to my skilled team, in particular, Carmel Finnegan for editing this work and Karen Murphy for collating the images.

Finally, life is too short not to do something we love. I have been surrounded by my precious children, Fleur and Tim, and special friends for a very long time. The enrichment they bring to my life is almost equalled by that amazing feeling one gets when a patient smiles back, with their confidence renewed and their eye contact back on line. I will continue to campaign, for the rest of my life, for two passions:

The right to see, the end of needless blindness. In 2018, we now have the technology; support www.righttosight.com.

The right to be seen as who we think we are and how we think we look. Much cosmetic work is actually rehabilitative and restorative; it should not only be in the demesne of the few who can afford it.

See better, look better, feel better.

Kate Coleman BSc, PhD, FRCS, FRCOphth
Blackrock Clinic
Dublin, Ireland

The first edition of this book was written in 2003, when the world was just awakening to the possibilities of botulinum toxin. Since then, it has become a billion-dollar industry, and rightly so. Fifty-five percent of indications for botulinum toxin injections are noncosmetic. It changes lives and makes them more bearable, particularly in patients following stroke and accidents who incur severe, unremitting spasm.

In the early days of oculoplastic surgery, we had to excise the orbicularis oculi muscle to allow a patient with severe blepharospasm to walk, to see. Since the mid-1980s, these patients have been well corrected with botulinum toxin injections, albeit regularly.

Management of aberrant signalling in the facial muscles of our patients has provided us with a wealth of information on neuromodulation and facial symmetry. This is the complex side of predicting the redirection of muscle signalling, once it is interfered with using botulinum toxin. This new edition brings 30 years of experience to these lessons in the hope of transferring the intuitive art to a new generation of managers of facial expression.

The goal of our patient treatments is to:
- Reconstruct
- Rehabilitate
- Refresh
- Restore
- Rejuvenate

The art is to always make the patient look like they have not interfered with their face, to look natural and to look, above all, normal and healthy.

This edition emphasises skills training to free the mind to be intuitive, to grasp the natural asymmetry most patients have and to move and respond with varying doses accordingly. It again emphasises the range of solutions which must be considered for a patient without always assuming that botulinum toxin is the answer. This approach works.

The evidence is here: photos of patients from the first edition, looking as natural and graceful 15 years later.

Never underestimate the gift you give your patients when you give them quiet confidence in their natural appearance; they look better, but most of all, they feel better. Normal people want to look normal.

The art of good botulinum treatment is always to make the patient look better, but not necessarily younger.

CONTENTS

CHAPTER 1

Historical Background

The *Clostridium* family of bacteria, common to most environments, produces spores that, on germination, release some of the deadliest toxins known to mankind. *Clostridium Perfringens* contaminates wounds and caused the infamous gas gangrene of World War 1; *Clostridium botulinum* produces botulinum toxin (BTX)—a powerful neurotoxin.

Clostridium botulinum was first identified in 1897, in Belgium, by Professor Emile van Ermengenen, who was investigating fatal cases of food poisoning following the consumption of macerated ham. It was named after the disease it causes, botulism, a lethal form of food poisoning originally associated with sausage meat (botulus is Latin for sausage). In the same year, an antiserum for botulism was made.

There are seven known serotypes of BTX (A, B, C, D, E, F and G). Serotypes A, B and E cause the classic foodborne disease with a flaccid paralysis of motor and autonomic nerves. Type B was first discovered in 1910, and the isolation of type A began in the 1920s. During the Second World War, research continued into this potent neurotoxin as a possible agent ('agent X') for biological warfare. Most of this work was carried out at the chemical warfare laboratories of Fort Detrick, Maryland, and Porton Down in the United Kingdom. Porton Chemicals was bought by Ipsen Pharmaceuticals in 1989 and is the source of Dysport.

Dr Alan Scott, an ophthalmologist from the Smith-Kettlewell Eye Research Foundation, became interested in substances that caused transient muscular paralysis. He acquired BTX type A from Fort Detrick and performed the first clinical tests on humans in 1978. His results in the treatment of strabismus (an abnormal contraction of the extraocular eye muscles) were published in 1982 and led to the extensive use of BTX type A by ophthalmologists in the treatment of blepharospasm (an abnormal twitching and contraction of the muscles around the eye), hemifacial spasm and cervical dystonia.

By the late 1980s, the author, an oculofacial and ophthalmic surgeon in Ireland, as well as colleagues in Canada and the United Kingdom, were each exploring different doses and methods for using BTX. The author worked on patients with facial asymmetry, especially Bell palsy, to calculate the doses required to 'balance' the innervation of the whole face.

Thereafter the story is well known. With good medical training and the correct selection of patients, BTX can be given easily, safely and repeatedly. There have been relatively few reported side effects despite ever-increasing demand in increasingly large doses, in particular for large muscle dystonia and spasm.

Thanks to Dr Scott, many lives have been enhanced and many more made bearable by this deadliest of poisons and astonishingly precise drug.

CHAPTER 2

Botulinum Toxin: Mode of Action and Serotypes

Dr. Kate Coleman, BSc PhD FRCS FRCOphth

A working knowledge of the pharmacology of botulinum toxin (BTX) is essential to understand the contraindications and complications of treatment with it.

Botulinum neurotoxins are metalloprotease polypeptides, comprising a protein molecule (150 Kd), which can be cleaved enzymatically into a heavy (H) (100 Kd) and a light (L) (50 Kd) chain (Fig. 2.1). These chains are normally held together by a disulphide bond, which is heat labile. Disruption of this bond inactivates the neurotoxin. This explains why BTX must be stored at the correct temperature and reconstituted carefully, preserving the integrity of the two-chained molecule. Prior to reconstitution, characteristics of Incobotulinum toxin A (Xeomin) reflect the lack of a complexing protein with the neurotoxin, allowing lpng term stability and reduced immunogenicity.

BTX induces paralysis by blocking the release of acetylcholine at the skeletal alpha motor neurone neuromuscular junction, thereby inhibiting the transmission of nerve impulses across the synaptic junction to the motor end plate.

> **USER TIP**
>
> Always consider possible central, as well as obvious peripheral, changes to the injected muscle following treatment (neuromodulation).

Muscular Contraction: Normal Cholinergic Transmission (Fig. 2.2)

Voluntary muscle contraction is a response to stimulation by action potentials passing along a nerve to the muscle. Once these action potentials reach a synapse at the neuromuscular junction, they stimulate an influx of calcium into the cytoplasm of the nerve ending. This increase in

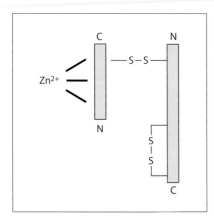

Fig. 2.1 Diagram of botulinum toxin molecule showing heavy and light chains. (From Aoki R. The development of Botox—its history and pharmacology. *Pain Digest.* 1998;8:337–341. With permission from Springer-Verlag.)

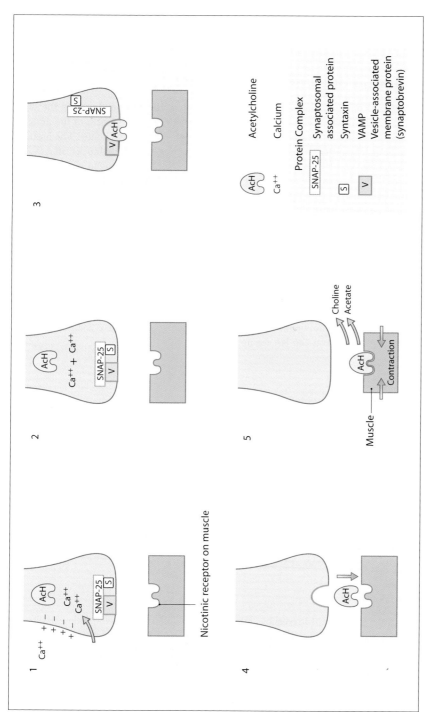

Fig. 2.2 Normal cholinergic transmission: (1) A signal passes down the cholinergic nerve, causing calcium to pass through the depolarising presynaptic membrane. (2) The calcium then triggers the binding of the acetylcholine molecule to a protein membrane complex. (3) The protein membrane complex allows the acetylcholine to pass into the synaptic cleft. (4) The acetylcholine travels across the synapse to a nicotinic receptor on the muscle, where it stimulates contraction before disintegrating into acetate and choline (5). *VAMP*, Vesicle-associated membrane protein.

calcium concentration allows acetylcholine to fuse with the membrane, using a protein complex, before crossing the synapse and fusing with nicotinic receptors on the muscle fibre. The protein complex consists of three types of protein: vesicle-associated membrane protein (VAMP; synaptobrevin), synaptosomal-associated protein (SNAP)-25 and syntaxin.

Mode of Action of Botulinum Toxin (Fig. 2.3)

Acetylcholine depends on a protein complex for its release from the nerve ending into the synapse. BTX, using a specific enzyme in the L-chain, interacts with one component of the protein complex of the nerve terminal, thereby inhibiting the discharge of the acetylcholine. The protein attacked is specific to the different serotypes of BTX; for example BTX-A blocks SNAP-25, whereas BTX-B blocks VAMP. BTX-B acts on a different cytoplasmic protein complex. The secretion of acetylcholine is disrupted when the L-chain of the BTX-B molecule cleaves a protein called synaptobrevin, also known as VAMP. Clinical trials have shown BTX-B to be effective for the treatment of patients with cervical dystonia, including those resistant to BTX-A.

Both the H- and L-chains of the BTX molecule are needed to block the release of acetylcholine. The H-chain attaches the BTX to the nerve membrane, allowing the L-chain to be transported to its site of action—the protein complex. The L-chain enzyme then cleaves the protein specific to the particular neurotoxin. Neuromuscular transmission ceases, and the target muscle atrophies reversibly.

AUTONOMIC ACTION

BTX also blocks autonomic cholinergic receptors. The duration of action is longer than for skeletal nerve endings, and effects can last for up to 12 months.

CENTRAL ACTION

BTX affects the gamma motor neurone, reducing muscle spindle afferent input to the central nervous system, and at high doses has been shown to reach the brain. Functional magnetic resonance imaging has shown that glabellar injections of BTX have resulted in functional uncoupling of brain stem centres with the amygdala. Other studies have confirmed reduction in the size of areas of basal ganglia in response to high-dose injections for spasticity. These central effects help to explain how BTX can ameliorate pain and chronic migraine, as well as supporting some studies suggesting improvement of depression. Studies have demonstrated retrograde and anterograde axonal transport along the branches of nociceptive neurones following peripheral nerve blockade. Pain relief has been shown to start prior to paralysis, outlasting the duration of the paralysis, supporting a noncholinergic mechanism. The antinociceptive effect is mediated by blockade of neuropeptides and inflammatory mediator release. There is evidence of inhibition of plasma membrane exposure of pain sensors at the peripheral level.

MUSCLE RECOVERY

Cleavage of the protein complex is irreversible, but the changes following BTX include a proliferation of axonal nerve buds to the target muscle and the regeneration of muscle end plates. New nerves 'bud' out across the motor endplates, albeit with irregularly spread cholinergic receptors

Muscle function takes between 24 hours and 5 days to cease; in contrast, recovery takes from 6 weeks with rimabotulinumtoxin B (Neurobloc) and an average of 14 weeks with onabotulinumtoxin A (Botox), Incobotulinumtoxin A (Xeomin) and abobotulinumtoxin B (Dysport). In the author's experience, duration of effect is dose and location dependent. Some muscles, the frontalis in particular, remain paralysed in some patients for as long as 5 months, after only one

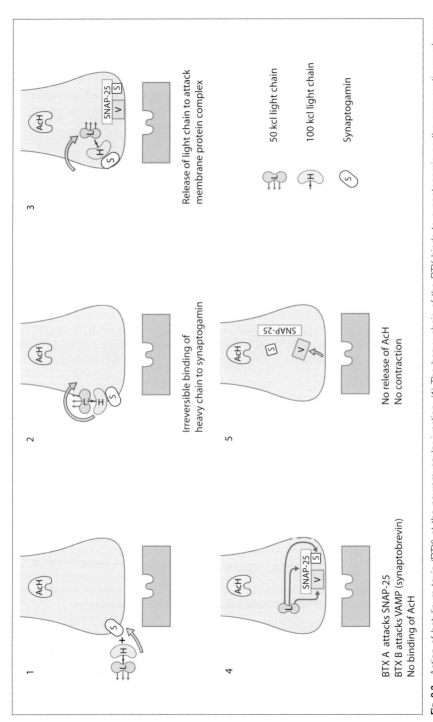

Fig. 2.3 Action of botulinum toxin (BTX) at the neuromuscular junction: (1) The heavy chain of the BTX binds to synaptogamin on the presynaptic membrane. (2) The heavy chain/synaptogamin complex enables the BTX light chain to enter the cell. (3) The light chain attacks the membrane complex and disables it so that NO ACETYLCHOLINE (AcH) BINDS. (4) BTX-A attacks the SNAP-25 protein of the membrane protein complex, and BTX-B attacks VAMP (synaptobrevin). (5) There is no release of AcH. *SNAP,* Synaptoscmal-associated protein; *VAMP,* vesicle-associated membrane protein.

treatment. Prolonged paralysis results in muscle atrophy, which has been shown to last years in the forehead musculature. There is also a suggestion of long-term reduction in central voluntary control, 'breaking the frown habit', as evidenced by other basal ganglia imaging studies following BTX-A administration.

The orbicularis oculi muscle requires 3 to 6 months to recover its function, but, even then, the muscle returns to only 70% to 80% of its original bulk. This explains the fact that even an isolated treatment can help the 'crow's feet' of patients who are reluctant to engage in a series of treatments.

USER TIP

Choose your dose to modify the desired duration of action.

IMMUNOGENICITY

The development of antibodies to one serotype does not preclude an effective response to another one. Reports suggest an incidence of 2% rate of antibody formation with serotype A (onabotulinumtoxin A, BOTOX) as opposed to 20% to 40% with serotype B (rimabotulinum toxin B, Myobloc). Research suggests that the production of these antibodies is related to the protein load of the neurotoxin. This has led to the development of incobotulinumtoxin A, Xeomin/Bocouture, with its free 150-kD molecule and no haemagglutinin complexing. The original Onabotulinumtoxin A (Botox) contained 25mg Protein/100units. The more recent Botox preparations have a reduced protein load of only 5mg/100units in comparison.

Immunogenicity has been linked to the frequency of administration of BTX and to its concentration. Ideally, therefore, good therapy should be spaced at a minimum of 12-week intervals and should use the lowest concentration effective for the desired duration of action.

Serotypes

There are seven serotypes of BTX, five of which are effective at the human neuromuscular junction (BTX-A, B, E, F and G). The different serotypes act by cleaving different proteins at the presynaptic vesicle.

Four types of BTX are currently licensed and available commercially in Europe and the United States (Table 2.1); three are BTX serotype A: Botox/Botox Cosmetic (onabotulinumtoxin A), Dysport/Azzalure (abobotulinumtoxin A) and Xeomin/Bocouture (incobotulinumtoxin A). Neurobloc/Myobloc is BTX type B. Several types of BTX-A have been emerging in other countries, some also from the HALL strain of BTX (e.g. Meditox, South Korea).

Concern must be highlighted about unlicensed online availability of poorly regulated toxins from other countries, including 'copies' of Allergan BOTOX with no toxin in the bottles. The author had experience with a toxin being launched in the Middle East, which caused local

TABLE 2.1 ■ **Botulinum Toxin Currently Licensed and Available Commercially in Europe and the United States**

BTX-A	BTX-A	BTX-A	BTX-B
Abobotulinumtoxin A	Incabotulinumtoxin A	Onabotulinumtoxin A	Rimabotulinumtoxin B
Dysport	Xeomin	Botox	Neurobloc
Azzalure	Bocouture	Vistabel	Myobloc

BTX, Botulinum toxin.

permanent muscle atrophy and scarring when injected. Other adverse reports include four cases of botulism in Florida due to toxic levels of BTX in unlicensed vials. The author currently uses only Dysport/Azzalure, Botox and Xeomin and will refer to these products and their differences in the rest of this manual.

USER TIP

Botulinum toxin acts by blocking release of acetylcholine from the nerve terminal.

USER TIP

Conditions and/or drugs affecting the nerve/muscle junction could also affect the botulinum toxin results.

CHAPTER 3

Clinical Indications and Use

The cosmetic indications for botulinum toxin have not changed since the first edition of this book and are listed in Box 3.1, but the noncosmetic indications now represent 55% of all botulinum toxin use. In the author's oculofacial practice, botulinum toxin is an essential first-line treatment for hemifacial and blepharospasm, post–facial nerve palsy synkinesis, chronic migraine, frontal 'trigeminal' headaches and hyperhidrosis. Table 3.1 provides a list of other uses at the time of press.

Much has been published on the differences between the different products, and the reader is referred to an excellent 2018 review on the same by Dr. Richard Glogau.

> **USER TIP**
>
> DIFFUSION is influenced by concentration, by product and by the concentration of receptors on the muscle being injected. More receptors mean less diffusion per volume injected.

BOX 3.1 ■ Cosmetic Indications For Botulinum Toxin

Crow's feet (periocular rhytids)	Pebbly chin
Vertical (glabellar) frown	Nasolabial folds
Horizontal (frontalis) frown	Jaw line (platysma)
Wrinkles on nose	Venus rings (horizontal neck rhytids)
Upper lip rhytids	Turkey neck (vertical platysma bands)
Vermilion border	Décolleté
Angle of mouth	Scar management

TABLE 3.1 ■ Noncosmetic Indications for Botulinum Toxin

Movement Disorders	Internal Organs	Other
Focal dystonias	Detrusor muscle	Hyperhidrosis
Essential tremor	Bladder spasm pain	Chronic migraine
Parkinsonism	Urinary retention	Tension headaches
Spasticity	Hyperactive/overactive	Trigeminal neuralgia
Post-stroke spasticity	Pelvic floor pain	Temporomandibular pain
Traumatic spasticity	Anal fissures	Spinal muscle pain
Multiple sclerosis	Benign prostate hyperplasia	Frey's syndrome
Eye movement disorders		Sialorrhoea

TABLE 3.2 ■ Botulinum Toxin Serotype Type A

Onabotulinumtoxin A	Abobotulinumtoxin A	Incobotulinumtoxin A
BOTOX/visabel	Dysport/Azzalure	Xeomin/Bocouture
900-kDa complex	<900 kDa	150 kDa
Vacuum-dried powder	Freeze-dried powder	Freeze-dried powder
2–8°	2–8°	Room temperature
HSA 500 μg	HSA 125 μg	HSA 1000 μg
NaCl (900 μg/vial)	Lactose (2.5 mg/vial)	Sucrose (4.7 mg/vial)
BOTOX: 100-U or 200-U vial	Dysport: 300 U or 500 U	Xeomin: 100 U or 200 U
Vistabel: 50 U	Azzalure: 125 U	Bocouture: 50 U
5 ng/100 U	4.35 ng/500 U	0.44 ng/100 U

Concentrations

Botulinum toxin is the most potent toxin known to mankind. It functions at very low concentrations and so can be assessed accurately only in terms of lethal dose unit per Swiss-Webster mouse. (Research is ongoing in to cell-based potency assay.) Different serotype A brands are shown in Table 3.2. One mouse unit (mu) is the median intraperitoneal dose required to kill 50% (LD_{50}) of a batch of 18- to 20-g female Swiss-Webster mice over 3 to 4 days.

The types of mice used by different producers differ and so the units discussed are NOT interchangeable. One vial of onabotulinumtoxin A (BOTOX, Fig. 3.1) contains 100 mu, while one vial of abobotulinumtoxin A (Dysport, Fig. 3.2) contains 500 'Speywood' mu. One vial of Xeomin (Fig. 3.3) contains 100 mu, similar to the BOTOX units assay. This variability of assay, coupled with the absence of a definitive human assay, means that the doses used have to be based

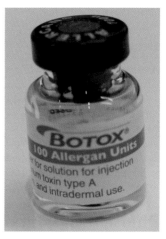

Fig. 3.1 Bottle of BOTOX.

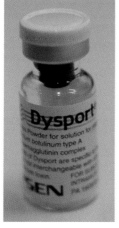

Fig. 3.2 Bottle of Dysport.

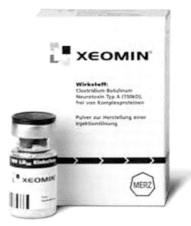

Fig. 3.3 Bottle of Xeomin.

on clinical experience. The three different products have different licences for use for different countries. Each has a cosmetic use licence for a smaller vial of the same product: BOTOX (Vistabel 50 U), Dysport (Azzalure 125 U) and Xeomin (Bocouture 50 U). (The author uses only botulinum toxin type A serotypes and refers only to these in this book.)

Clinical efficacy is directly related to the degree of dilution of the toxin, the muscle targeted, and the volume injected. Botulinum toxin adheres to the muscle receptor, and the diffusion will be greater for fewer receptors than for more per site.

In a cosmetic practice, different outcomes require different combinations of onset, duration and diffusion of effect. The art is to learn how to use the combinations of the available products to 'mould' the tone of the area being treated.

> **USER TIP**
>
> A beginner should use one botulinumtoxin A to start, at one dilution, for all treatments and learn to change the volume and site of injection to get predictable results.

Onset of Effect

A consensus of clinical experience suggests onset may be as early as day 2 and usually before day 6 with all three products.

Early onset of effect is desirable for certain 'special occasions' but usually most wanted when correcting an unpredicted facial muscle movement. This will be discussed in Chapters 6 to 10, but for example, if a patient experiences an alarming brow 'peak', a top-up to the offending muscle, with effect as soon as possible, is strongly desired. The author chooses abobotulinumtoxin A (Azzalure), which often becomes active, depending on the patient, on day 2.

In general, treatments are planned with the patient, knowing that the effect will take up to 5 days to appear and then the following 7 to 10 days to 'balance out'. This works for all three products.

Diffusion and Duration

Dilutions and resulting unit per volume are shown in Tables 3.3 and 3.4.

BOTOX and Xeomin behave with similar unit-per-vial potency. The potency of one 100 U vial of BOTOX is not the same as that of one 500 U vial of Dysport. Several studies suggest that 3 to 5 units of Dysport/Azzalure equate with 1 unit of BOTOX.

Both incabotulinumtoxin A (Xeomin) and onabotulinumtoxin A (BOTOX) have similar durations of action, their effects wearing off after 12 to 14 weeks. Clinical trials have compared diffusion properties, a theory being that a small protein complex could diffuse further, but results suggest equal diffusion 'per equivalent dosage'. The studies referred to used a ratio of 1:4 onabotulinumtoxin A (BOTOX) to abobotulinumtoxin A (Azzalure/Dysport).

TABLE 3.3 ■ Concentration of BOTOX/Xeomin per Dilution With Preservative-Free Normal Saline

BOTOX/Xeomin Units Per 0.1 mL	BOTOX/Xeomin 100 IU Add	BOTOX/Xeomin 50 IU Add
10 units	1 mL	0.5 mL
4 units	2.5 mL	1.25 mL
3.3 units	3 mL	1.5 mL
3.5 units	3.5 mL	1.75 mL
4 units	4 mL	2 mL

TABLE 3.4 ■ Concentration of Dysport/Azzalure With Preservative-Free Normal Saline

Dysport/Azzalure Units Per 0.1 mL	Dysport 500 Units Add	Azzalure 125 Units Add
50	1 mL	0.25 mL
20	2.5 mL	0.625 mL
16.66	3 mL	0.75 mL
14.3	3.5 mL	0.875 mL
12.5	4 mL	1 mL

The author often uses a stronger equivalent dose ratio of ≥1:3.5. Azzalure appears to diffuse to more muscle fibres per site of injection than BOTOX and appears to last longer at these equivalent concentrations. The author modifies the dilution if a shorter duration of action is required, as will be seen in Chapters 6 to 10.

The protein content of the botulinumtoxin A complex is sometimes cited as a reason for choosing between the products. Incobotulinumtoxin A, Xeomin, has no haemagglutinin protein complexed with its 150-kDa botulinumtoxin A molecule and so is unlikely to have the same antigenic properties as other preparations. This may be relevant in large doses, for example with cervical dystonia, but does not seem relevant to date with rejuvenation doses.

The protein content of BOTOX has changed since it was introduced to Europe in 1989. The original batch, from Dr. Scott's company Oculinum, of 150 g of pure crystallised toxin, was prepared by Dr. Schantz in 1979. BOTOX is a vacuum-dried form of purified botulinumtoxin A, produced by cultures of the Hall strain of *Clostridium botulinus*. It is isolated as a crystalline protein complex from the culture solution by a series of acid preparations and then redissolved in a solution containing saline and albumin. It is then filtered using a sterile technique before vacuum drying. This author's experience with onabotulinumtoxin A (BOTOX) from 1989 to 1997 was with the original Schantz preparation. In 1997, a new batch was prepared by Allergan with different labelling. This batch, in current use, contains 20% less protein than the original one and so is less likely to stimulate an albumin-related allergic response. The author has seen no cases of immunogenicity to onabotulinumtoxin A (BOTOX) since 1997.

- *Onabotulinumtoxin A (BOTOX) is produced by a precipitation technique and freeze-dried to a powder.*
- *Incabotulinumtoxin A (Xeomin) is a freeze-dried powder.*
- *Abobotulinumtoxin A (Azzalure/Dysport) is produced by column-based purification and freeze-dried to a powder.*
- *Rimabotulinumtoxin B (Myobloc) is a high-molecular-weight botulinumtoxin B that is not lyophilised but a buffered intact protein complex in liquid form, at a pH of 5.5.*

Economics

An experienced practitioner with a busy botulinumtoxin A practice may choose among the three on economic grounds only—all are currently available at the same price in Ireland. Studies in management of dystonia have shown that Azzalure/Dysport, followed by Xeomin, followed by BOTOX were the most economical in Europe.

An inexperienced practitioner, with few patients and an irregular demand for botulinumtoxin A, may initially prefer the smaller vials of Azzalure, Vistabel and Bocouture.

It is not recommended to store botulinumtoxin A for more than 24 hours following reconstitution, but several studies support the author's long-term experience of at least 2-weeks efficacy when stored at correct temperatures without undue mechanical friction. Furthermore, colleagues report successful use of frozen reconstituted onabotulinumtoxin A (BOTOX) after 6 months.

CLINICAL USE GUIDELINES

Here are examples of how, in the author's clinic, the choice between products is generally made:

Diffusion (Fig. 3.4)

- For a small diffusion zone, one may use a concentrated solution, e.g. 1 mL NaCl added to 500 U abobotulinumtoxin A (Dysport) and inject 0.02 mL (i.e. 10 units); or a use a smaller volume of a more dilute solution, which will diffuse more deeply but have a shorter duration of action or the third option, which the author favours, is to use a concentrated solution of BOTOX or Xeomin (onabotulinumtoxin A), e.g., 0.025 mLs of 1 mL added to 100 units.
- For a large diffusion zone, use 3.5 mL/NaCl to 500 U abobotulinumtoxin A (Dysport) or 0.9 mL/NaCl to 125 U Azzalure and inject 0.1 mL. This will create a possible diffusion circle diameter of 3 cm.

USER TIP

DURATION may be reduced by increasing the dilution, or by placing more superficially on the muscle complex, or both.

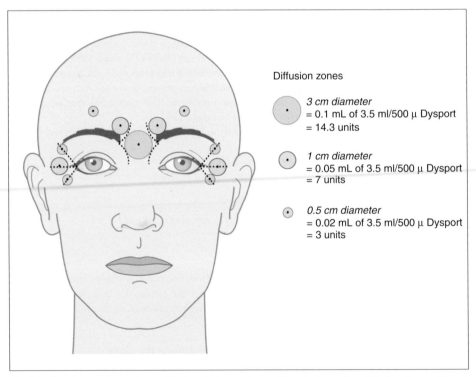

Diffusion zones

3 cm diameter
= 0.1 mL of 3.5 ml/500 µ Dysport
= 14.3 units

1 cm diameter
= 0.05 mL of 3.5 ml/500 µ Dysport
= 7 units

0.5 cm diameter
= 0.02 mL of 3.5 ml/500 µ Dysport
= 3 units

Fig. 3.4 Drawing to demonstrate diffusion circles of three different sizes when injecting three different volumes of abobotulinumtoxin A.

Duration

A short duration of action is ideal for new patients with unpredictable facial asymmetry, and those who are happier to know that if they are unhappy with the results of their treatment, that the effect will wear off after only 6 weeks, as opposed to over 12 weeks with the higher concentrations. They may be offered a 'top-up' then. It is also possible to get even shorter durations of action with further dilution of the dose. It is worth noting that inadequate storage of botulinumtoxin A (e.g. at an incorrect temperature), or excessive dilution, also shortens the duration of effect. Duration may be inadvertently reduced by agitating the bottle of botulinum toxin once it has been re-constituted.

For a longer duration, greater than 12 weeks, in a suitable site, increase the concentration of abobotulinumtoxin A (Azzalure) by adding less than 1 mL NaCl to the 125 U vial. NOTE that in our experience, the diffusion circle will be smaller for onabotulinumtoxin A and incobotulinumtoxin A, than for abobotulinumtoxin A, for the same volume of the same concentration.

The author has used Azzalure (abobotulinumtoxin A) since 1988 and BOTOX (onabotulinumtoxin A) since 1989, the choice depending on the site of injection. More recently, Xeomin (incobotulinumtoxin A) has become available and is also used as an alternative wherever BOTOX may be chosen. However, Neurobloc (rimabotulinumtoxin B) has a high protein load and 'stings', and the author has stopped using it for oculoplastic choices.

USER TIP

Think in volume/millilitre solution and not units/botulinum toxin A when injecting a patient. This allows good control and safety because one eye should always watch the volume scale gauge while injecting.

Patient Preparation and Injection Skills

Presentation

Botulinumtoxin A (BTX-A) vials have changed in size and shape over time. Specific instructions are readily available on the product websites and in the product insert packaging. Research is ongoing on the new liquid form of BTX-A, as well as topically applied preparations, but the three BTX-A products used by the author, onabotulinumtoxin A (onaBTX-A), incobotulinumtoxin A (incoBTX-A) and abobotulinumtoxin B (aboBTX-B), are presented as freeze-dried powder in a glass vial. The vials frequently look empty to the inexperienced eye because the powder tends to rest in their bottom angle (Fig. 4.1). The vials vary in size, depending on brand and quantity of units, and this will influence the capacity for filling with normal saline for more dilute preparations.

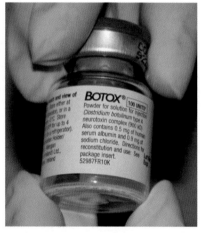

Fig. 4.1 Photograph of BOTOX vial showing powder at base prior to reconstitution.

There are strict guidelines for storage of botulinum toxin to prevent denaturation and maintain maximum efficacy. OnaBTX-A and aboBTX-A should be stored, before reconstitution, either frozen at −5°C or in a refrigerator at 2°C to 8°C until reconstituted. IncoBTX-A may be stored at room temperature, up to 25°C, until reconstituted. Once reconstituted, they all must be stored at 2°C to 8°C (refrigeration temperature). A thermos flask or a vaccination transporter may be used to maintain the solution at 2°C to 8°C if a refrigerator is not available in the clinic.

Reconstitution

It is recommended that all products are reconstituted with preservative-free normal saline, which is what the author routinely uses. Several studies have shown successful reconstitution with preserved normal saline, with reports of 48% more comfort when compared with preservative-free saline. Some studies have included 0.5% xylocaine to improve comfort.

The rubber seal on the vial should be wiped with an alcohol swab before using a 5-mL syringe to inject the desired volume of normal preservative-free saline. A green 25-gauge needle is inserted carefully through the centre of the bung, but care must be taken with BOTOX bungs, which can freeze solid. The needle can easily enter at an angle, releasing pieces of rubber into the solution.

USER TIP

Never agitate botulinum toxin solution when reconstituting it. It will not work!

The product is vacuum-sealed. If no pull on the plunger is felt, then the vial must be discarded. Air can be injected into the vial to avoid too rapid a reconstitution, and a thumb can be placed under the plunger of the syringe to control the rate of release of saline onto the powder (Fig. 4.2). The saline must not gush in and agitate the solution mechanically. This will denature it by disrupting the delicate disulphide bonds. Studies have confirmed that it will still be effective but with a curtailed duration of effect. Rotating the vial during injection, and gently swirling the solution, will capture any powder trapped in the 'lid' part of the vials, especially with incoBTX-A (Xeomin/Bocouture).

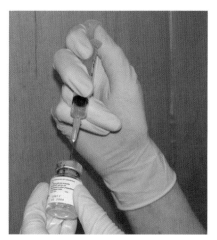

Fig. 4.2   Controlled reconstitution.

Injection

We recommend using no bigger than 1 mL tuberculin or insulin syringes. These are essential for the dose to be gauged accurately during injection. The doses recommended in this book are given in units of volume. The finest mark on a 1-mL syringe is 0.01: we often recommend using 0.025 mL and 0.01 mL (more later). Beginners may prefer a 0.05-mL syringe. Constant practice with 0.5-mL insulin syringes and then 1-mL syringes (Fig. 4.3) will develop the sense of touch to repeatedly administer small 'droplets' if necessary. The author prefers to use a 1-mL syringe and often more than one 30-gauge needle to keep the needle sharp while minimising stimulation of the nociceptors on the skin surface.

USER TIP

Always watch the gauge of the syringe while injecting to be certain of the volume you are injecting.

Transport

BTX-A can be transported after reconstitution if the solution is not agitated. Ideally it should be reconstituted after the journey; agitation denatures the toxin and greatly reduces its duration of action

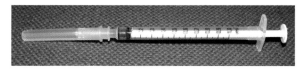

Fig. 4.3   One-millilitre syringe.

Aspiration

Always use gloves for self-protection. The solution should be aspirated freshly for each patient, although some doctors recommend preaspiration of BTX-A in several 1-mL syringes, and then storing them in the refrigerator. Manufacturers recommend a single vial per patient, which must be used within 4 hours of reconstitution.

Botulinum toxin is potent and very expensive, so each drop must be used to its maximum effect. Even an injection as small as 0.01 mL is effective in certain sites.

Take care to remove the 25-gauge needle from the bottle after aspiration, particularly with Dysport, where the combination of a small vial and a viscous solution encourages seepages from the needle.

Once aspiration is complete, attach a 30-gauge needle to the hub of the syringe. Take care that the batches of needles and syringes fit well together, and beware of attachments so loose that the toxin dribbles from the hub during injection. This is wasteful and may be hazardous if the leaked fluid contacts the patient's face (ingestion of botulinum toxin droplets has been suspected of causing mild gastroenteritis). Clear the air bubble from the syringe using minimal agitation. This requires more care with Dysport/Azzalure because of its greater viscosity.

> **USER TIP**
>
> Wipe away any spilled botulinum toxin with a hypochlorite solution

Skill must be acquired to confidently be able to administer the lowest number of BTX units at the highest concentration (i.e. a very small volume of solution) repeatedly and accurately. It is easy to administer a dilute solution of the same units at a larger volume.

Injection Technique

Good injection technique is critical for such a powerful agent because it takes a trained light touch to inject a tiny dose. Very few chemicals continue to be effective at such high dilutions. There is a real art to being able to manipulate the combination of extremely low with normal and high doses in the one treatment. The injections for rejuvenation are being administered to a continuum of facial muscle fibres. To be confident of offering aesthetically optimal treatment, the user must be skilled with injection technique. Once a single muscle tone is altered with a primary BTX-A injection, there is an immediate adaptation by both surrounding muscles, as well as remote 'paired' and contralateral muscles. Very small doses are excellent at controlling the secondary BTX-A effect. The user must be adept at injecting intradermally, subcutaneously, intramuscularly, giving small and large doses and, most of all, observing and avoiding arteries, veins and nerves.

The injector must know how to gauge the journey of the needle through the skin and muscle at different sites on the face and neck. This is a sense of touch which can be acquired only with practice.

Skill Development

Practise:
1. Entering the skin to create the least amount of pain
2. Entering the skin and muscle to the correct depth
3. Delivering the expected 'circle of diffusion' of toxin per volume injected.

PAIN

Topical anaesthesia makes little difference to the pain of intramuscular injections, unless highly concentrated (e.g. LMX) or in place long enough to penetrate. SLOW insertion of the needle makes a big difference to the perception of pain. The goal is to enter the skin without causing it to 'dip' and stimulate the pain receptors on either side (Fig. 4.4). It helps to enter at a 90 degree angle to the surface because that is the smallest surface area stimulated. With practice, it is actually possible to 'get lucky', to enter in between the pain receptors with the patient feeling nothing.

PRACTISE CIRCLES OF DIFFUSION

Fill a 1-mL syringe with coloured water (the author uses fluorescein) and attach a 30-gauge needle.
Use a wad of thick absorbent paper (e.g. four sheets of thickest kitchen roll).
Use coins or a compass to draw circles ranging from 0.5 cm to 2 cm (some paper comes
    preprinted with suitable shapes).
Practise placing the 30-gauge needle tip just under the first ply of the absorbent paper and repeat-
    edly filling the exact circles with coloured fluid.
To do this, the injector must inject the exact centre of the circle, injecting an identical volume
    repeatedly to fill a specific circle size (Fig. 4.5).

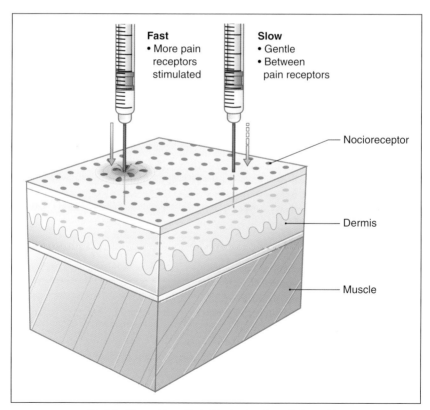

Fig. 4.4 Pin cushion effect of fast entry of needle in to skin.

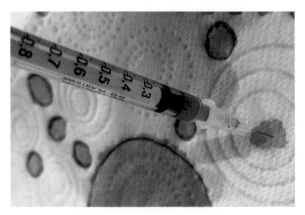

Fig. 4.5   Creating diffusion circles of different sizes.

CIRCLES OF VOLUME

Once practised, focus on carefully watching the syringe mark while injecting precise volumes of coloured water in to a wad of blank absorbent paper.

Practise 0.1-mL circles

Practise 0.05-mL circles

Practise 0.025-mL circles

Practise 0.01-mL 'drops' circles

Patient Skills

The injection practice should now have developed an instinctive sense of 'volume = circle size'.

The dosages in this book are taught as 'volumes'.

With practice, the injector can look at a muscle, decide on the 'size of circle' of BTX-A needed and choose the volume to provide that dose for the specific muscle.

It will become intuitive, second nature, to inject varying amounts, with an eye on the volume scale, to the various muscles to 'shape' the result.

The volumes will be suggested in Chapters 8 to 10.

NEXT STEPS: HOW TO INJECT A PATIENT

From now on, examine every patient to calculate where to place which sized circles. The injection will go in to a dot drawn at the centre of each circle.

As the face is examined, try to visualise the 'circles' of coloured water overlapping the muscles to be relaxed. Decide if a circle size is too close to relaxing the wrong part of a muscle, and move the circle centre, for example, to a higher place for a higher injection site. Visualise the different coloured circles fitting over the muscles to be relaxed, and then make sure that there is no unnecessary overlap with areas to be avoided or adequate overlap with areas to be treated (Fig. 4.6).

Focus on acquiring a 'feeling' of volume equilibrating with 'effect on the muscle'. This is akin to a sense of injecting circles of paint under the skin. Injecting a bigger volume will give a sense of reaching and relaxing a bigger surface area. This 'feeling' is an actual physical sensation of more or less pressure on the syringe as one injects larger or smaller volumes.

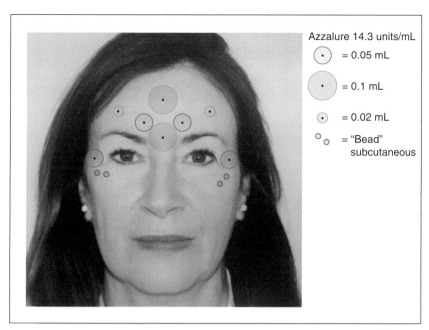

Fig. 4.6 Visualise adjacent diffusion circles over the treatment zones.

Avoid initially focussing on delivering 'units', as with many guides, because the delivery of units will not parallel the area of muscle treated visually with pressure on the syringe. It means that the injector does not have to constantly remember the number of units per dilution, just observe different volume marks on the syringe. An excellent result can be achieved by using different volumes of the same concentration (e.g. dilute a 100-U vial of onaBTX A [BOTOX] with 1 mL) for all initial treatments until confidence has developed.

'STARTER' PATIENTS

Start with a fixed concentration of BTX-A, and select only patients for whom this is appropriate.

It is very helpful to get practice giving 0.05-mL volume to patients who are having `Grid' treatments of the same volume. For example:

- Neck treatments for thin subdermal injections
- Hyperhidrosis treatments for deeper intradermal 'blebs' of 0.05 mL
- Chronic migraine treatments for deep intrascalp 0.05-mL injections.

It is also good to start on patients having treatment for bilateral blepharospasm, taking great care to develop a sense of difference between the needle entering the thicker orbital orbicularis muscle versus the paper-thin lower pretarsal orbicularis and, lastly, the very thin upper preseptal orbicularis under the medial brow. This is where diffusion to the upper levator muscle is most likely to happen, yet the area must often be treated to reduce disabling spasm. Raise the skin here with the needle tip and administer 0.0125 mL subcutaneously.

Beginners should not induce PTOSIS by avoiding the following cosmetic low-volume treatments (<0.05 mL) until skilled:

- Any glabellar treatments to patients with low heavy eyebrows, because these require a high concentration of BTX in a low volume to prevent excursion to the anterior levator muscle complex and ptosis.

■ Any attempt at 'brow lifts' which require small volumes to the brow depressors lateral to the lateral orbital rim and inferior to the supero medial orbital rims.

Once comfortable with the sense of volume and distribution (circle size), in particular administering 0.0125 and 0.025 mL volumes, then it is safe to prepare more concentrated solutions of BTX and address more difficult areas with impunity.

USER TIP

Larger volume will cause larger diffusion.
Higher concentration will cause less diffusion.

Patient Preparation

An inexperienced worker should mark the injection sites with a washable skin marker or pale sharp brow pencil, having first wiped the sites with an alcohol swab. It is important to sterilise the skin at the injection site because many patients wear a make-up foundation. Local granulomas or erythematous nodules can develop at injection sites (Fig. 4.7), but the author has never seen areas of infection or cellulitis related to an injection. Some practitioners suggest that alcohol denatures the toxin. If this were so, then every injection site swabbed with alcohol during a treatment session should have a similar effect on the toxin at the time of injection. However, the author has seen no difference in the effect of BTX-A when given simultaneously to sites which have been swabbed (forehead) and have not (eye zone in patients who find alcohol too irritating and are simply swabbed with saline).

Botulinum toxin can be injected intramuscularly, subcutaneously and as a 'bleb' beneath the epidermis. However, most doses in this book are based on intramuscular injections and have been derived from experience with blepharospasm. Subcutaneous injections are highly effective but need more injection sites to allow for maximum absorption. Subepithelial 'blebs' are invaluable for smoothing out the superficial attachments of skin to the underlying muscle whilst continuing to maintain resting muscle tone. These are usually given in a higher dilution to allow greater diffusion between the surface of the muscle and the skin. The patient is advised that such treatments last for only 6 weeks as opposed to the full 12 weeks expected from intramuscular injections. Pretarsal orbicularis injections are usually given intramuscularly because the skin here is only 0.5 mm thick. Intramuscular placement stings less and produces less local erythema. However, it carries a slight risk of causing intramuscular bruising. In our clinic, we use intradermal injections for hyperhidrosis, some dermatitis and some migraine (scalp) treatments.

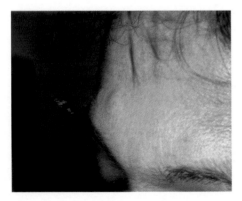

Fig. 4.7 Granuloma on the forehead from botulinum toxin injection.

Dosage

Each vial comes with recommended doses from the manufacturers of the product for treatment to the glabellar complex and the crow's feet area. A review of the literature provides information on the dosage preferences of a variety of practitioners. The author has validated the doses suggested in this book over the course of more than 30 years of treatments given since she herself, then a junior Ophthalmologist, started developing the cosmetic doses and uses in 1988. With experience, the reader should get a feeling for the required dose for each patient—and may well modify these doses accordingly. The following guidelines based on the author's experience may be useful:

Aim to use the smallest volume of the lowest concentration necessary to provide paralysis of the target muscle for at least 12 weeks.

Decide in advance how far you want the injection to diffuse (visualising the 'coloured circles from practice').

Remember that, on average, 4 units in 0.1 mL of BOTOX will diffuse 1 cm; 14.3 units of Dysport in 0.1 mL will diffuse 3 cm; 14.3 units of Dysport in 0.05 mL will diffuse less (approximately 1.5 cm), as will 2 units of BOTOX in 0.05 mL.

Select the injection site so that treatment will not extend beyond the desired diffusion zone, for example 0.1 mL of BOTOX injected 1 cm above the superior orbital rim (not brow) to treat the glabellar muscle. This avoids diffusion towards the levator muscle (Fig. 4.8). Likewise, inject 0.05 mL of Azzalure 1 cm from the lateral canthus (outer corner of the eyelid) to avoid diffusion medially.

Base your choice of dosage on the recommendations given in Chapters 7, 8 and 9. Most of your patients will receive the same dose for the same rhytids; but one aim of this book is to leave the reader with confidence in how to treat the unpredictable minority too.

USER TIP

Concentration of botulinum toxin:

Too weak = short duration of action
Too strong = risk of increased side effects

Choose larger diffusion circles for the following sites:
- Treatment of frontalis
- Extended treatment of crow's feet (inferolaterally over zygomatic arch)

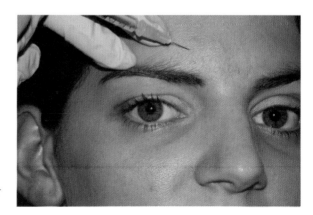

Fig. 4.8 Injecting at 1 cm over superior orbital area.

Choose smaller diffusion circles for the following sites:

- Lateral canthus
- Pre tarsal orbicularis
- Close to superior orbital rim

USER TIP

Increased volume dilution per unit botulinum toxin means increased diffusion.

USER TIP

Rough estimate: Add 3.5 mL to 500 units Dysport and expect:

14.3 units Dysport in 0.1 mL gives a 3-cm diffusion circle.
7 units Dysport in 0.05 mL gives a 1.5-cm diffusion circle.
3.5 units Dysport in 0.02 mL gives a 0.5-cm diffusion circle.

Patient Treatment

FRONTALIS ZONE

Ask the patient to frown while assessing the bulk of muscle contraction, then relax the patient and inject at the point noted. When injecting the forehead, gently tip the periosteum (sensitive) with the needle, withdraw slightly, and inject while watching the syringe gradations. With experience, one soon becomes familiar with the sensation of muscle bulk, and the periosteum is rarely touched. Take care to point the needle away from danger.

It is sometimes useful to hold the muscle site between two fingers, especially in the glabellar area (Fig. 4.9).

CROW'S FEET

Ask the patients to smile, note the centre point of movement, then ask them to relax. Mark the centres of expected circles of diffusion, then inject the centre (Fig. 4.10). Take care not to point the needle towards the orbital septum when injecting the lateral canthus.

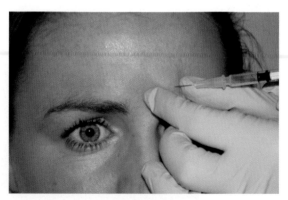

Fig. 4.9 Holding the muscle between the two fingers when injecting the glabella.

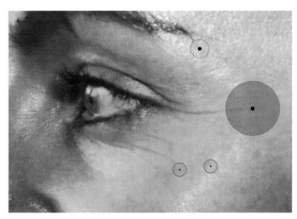

Fig. 4.10 Circles of diffusion in crow's feet treatment zone.

Post Injection

The patient should be asked to press on the site with a tissue immediately after the injection—even while other sites are being treated. This minimises bruising. Any bruising that occurs should be treated immediately with an ice pack from the freezer. Camouflage cream or make-up is then applied before the patient goes home.

Some experts recommend the avoidance of flying or lying down after treatment. This is supposed to reduce untoward diffusion and, hence, side effects such as ptosis. However, the author has had only one case of ptosis in more than 30 years of treatments and has seen no evidence to confirm this theory.

Time

An average botulinum appointment lasts a maximum of 10 minutes. This excludes the first counselling visit (often 90 minutes) but includes reading and signing the consent form, the injections and settling the account. A nurse practitioner may prepare the patient and provide information on other aspects of rhytid prevention and management, thus reducing the time spent with the practitioner.

USER TIP

Imagine that every time the needle pierces the skin, it is like pressing a soft pin cushion, so that the pins in it bend down towards each other. Now visualise the pins as pain receptors, which signal pain only if they move. Aim to enter with NO movement.

USER TIP

Avoid the supraorbital nerve, vein and artery complex when injecting the glabellar area. Study the anatomy and, if in doubt, feel for the supraorbital notch under the medial aspect of the brow.

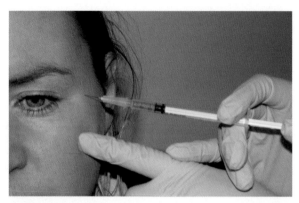

Fig. 4.11   Steady the injecting hand, and avoid sudden movement by the patient towards the needle.

USER TIP

Spread the lateral orbital skin between two fingers to observe the orbital veins clearly and take care to inject around these.

USER TIP

Steady the injecting hand by resting the little finger on the face while spreading the skin with the other hand. Look carefully for and avoid superficial veins (Fig. 4.11).

CHAPTER 5

Patient Selection: The Art of Understanding Neuromodulation and Symmetry

One of the most difficult things to do for a beginner with botulinum toxin (BTX) is to anticipate how the other muscles on the face will react if injections are given to a muscle. It is easy to see what happens when the treated muscle is paralysed but less easy to anticipate where the signal to 'that' muscle will now divert to.

It is also tempting to assume that a right and left muscle will require the same dose for the same amount of paralysis, but because of natural asymmetry, this does not always happen.

The art lies in learning how to predict where the signals will go after treatment and how to anticipate and prevent unwanted action of other muscles on the face.

It is important to have a deep understanding of this signalling to muscles of the face before interfering with the muscle tone of a patient's face and neck. Examples of muscle signal pairs are shown in Table 5.1.

Principles of Balancing the Face

- Think of BTX as blocking the innervation of a specific area of muscle, as opposed to blocking the whole muscle.
- Always try to guess where the innervation will go to instead, once you have blocked it, and anticipate extra movement elsewhere which might need treatment.
- Always remember the long-term effects you are creating via central control of innervation and feedback; this how you 'train' the muscles.

USER TIP

Never assume that both sides of the face receive equal innervation.

TABLE 5.1 ■ Paired Muscles of Expression

Muscle Action	Paired Muscle Action
Corrugator	Depressor anguli oris (sad)
Frontalis muscle	Mentalis (horror)
Frontalis muscle	Depressor anguli oris
Frontalis muscle	Orbicularis oculi
Frontalis muscle	Zygomaticus
Orbicularis oculi	Zygomaticus (smile)

Resting Tone

The muscles of the face tend to mirror each other.

Many wrongly forget that the muscles have a resting tone when not contracting and assume that the muscles are relaxed when the patient is not actively contracting them. A good way to demonstrate what the patient will look like after resting tone is turned off is to examine their eyebrows. When the brows are gently massaged downwards, with the patient's eyes shut, they often descend to a lower resting position. This is without resting tone. This is where they would 'live' if all their frontalis received BTX.

The basic nerve signal to a muscle of facial expression is usually from a tonically active neuron that is a cholinergic neuron that fires at 0.5 to 3 impulses per second during the entire duration of the stimulus. This allows the muscle to have a resting tone and to provide a baseline support to the facial structures in between voluntary facial movements. For example, the frontalis muscle of the forehead, innervated by the zygomaticofacial branch of the facial nerve VII, usually has a resting tone (Fig. 5.1A). The patient may raise the eyebrows on command by contracting the frontalis muscle (see Fig. 5.1B), but it is usually possible to 'relax' the resting tone and to bring the brows to a lower level than their normal resting tone (see Fig. 5.1C). This latter position imitates and thus demonstrates the unwanted result of too much BTX across the forehead in an unsuitable patient.

Voluntary and Involuntary Movement

Right and left muscle pairs tend to contract simultaneously. They may also be accompanied by relaxation of their antagonist muscles. Each muscle of the pair may have a different bulk in response to the size of the underlying bony framework

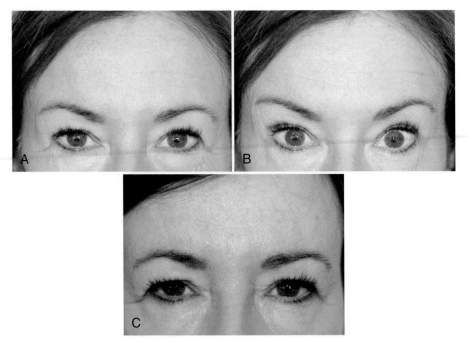

Fig. 5.1 Patient with **(A)** resting forehead tone, **(B)** raising eyebrows and **(C)** forced relaxation, demonstrating unwanted effect of too much botulinum toxin.

When a facial muscle is turned on to contract, its opposing antagonist muscle is turned off to relax. The levator muscle cannot open the eyelid unless the orbicularis muscle stops closing it, and vice versa.

A voluntary signal to the face (e.g. 'SMILE') can cause contraction of the right and left lateral orbicularis oculi (giving crow's feet), as well as elevation of the outer corners of the mouth (orbicularis oris), but ALSO relaxation of the opposing brow elevators (frontalis fibres) and mouth depressors (depressor anguli oris and depressor labii inferioris).

The concept of bilateral signalling to muscles on opposite sides of the face was first expressed by Ewald Hering in the 19th century when he espoused his theory of binocular vision. Hering's law is often referred to when describing how the extraocular muscles of the eyes work. For example, a gaze to the right side requires contraction of the right lateral rectus to pull the eye to the right and relaxation of the right medial rectus, whilst contracting the left medial rectus to pull the left eye in the same direction at the same time as the right, and relaxing the left lateral rectus. This reflex is so strong that an ophthalmic surgeon may correct an inward turning left eye, due to an overactive medial rectus, by operating to strengthen the opposing muscle on the other eye, the right lateral rectus.

The facial muscles are supplied by nerves which have their roots in the midbrain complex. Information on muscle tone is relayed through the midbrain and back to both sides of the face (Fig. 5.2).

Research into facial dystonias has confirmed supranuclear motor control of the paired muscle groups. This control is necessary for functions such as blinking, postural maintenance and extraocular muscle movements. Imaging modalities have shown that central control is relayed through the posterior commissure, rostral brainstem and the basal ganglia of the brain. The frontal cortex and cerebellum are also involved in neuromodulation. The size of the grey matter volume in the left parietal lobe had been observed to decrease in parallel to BTX treatment of spasticity. For example, variations in the contralateral blink reflex have been observed with ipsilateral facial nerve lesions.

It is believed that facial expression is produced by the branching pattern of the common–stem last order presynaptic input fibres innervating motor neurones supplying different muscles. Multiunit surface/electromyography recordings have demonstrated 'coding' of pairs. Voluntary command through the motor cortex can control expression and cocontraction through the facial nucleus subnuclei.

In the author's experience, patients who can 'wriggle their ears' have a very active galea aponeurotica–frontalis action. BTX to the frontalis redirects extra innervation to the scalp, and now, brow elevation creates a 'crumple' in the upper third of the forehead (see Chapter 8). However, the author has found that patients often have great difficulty wiggling their ears when their corrugators are manually 'blocked' to stop them pushing their eyebrows together! It appears that the glabellar complex is linked to the galea aponeurotica ear wriggling. This, of course, is what happens when a dog points its ears and draws its brows together when alerted (Fig. 5.3).

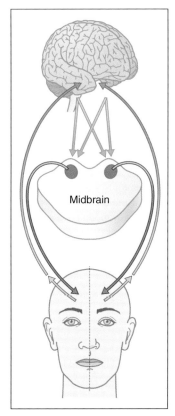

Fig. 5.2 Diagram demonstrating passage of signal from the muscle spindles through the brain and then to both sides of the face allowing simultaneous neuromodulation of bilateral muscle tone.

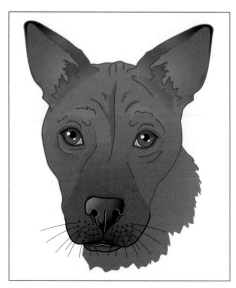

Fig. 5.3 Drawing demonstrating paired expression between glabella and scalp in an alert dog, contracting the glabella (eyebrows drawn together) and the scalp muscles simultaneously (ears raised).

Botulinum Toxin as a Powerful Neuromodulator

BTX will stop the release of Acetylcholine at a muscle, but in the author's experience, it never acts in isolation. There is almost always a perceptible change in the neighbouring innervated muscles and the paired muscles. There is also a central response, altering the impetus to signal the muscle with time.

In the early days of BTX, at the time of printing of the first edition of this book, it was not uncommon to see patients in the United States who had simply received the US Food and Drug Administration (FDA)-approved 'glabellar treatment', as printed on the BOTOX box leaflet, without any modulation of the rest of the forehead complex, because that had remained 'off label'. The bilateral sharp arched 'BOTOX brows' are currently seen only with inexperience when the injector does not take care to 'neutralise' the frontalis fibres, which will receive extra innervation, relayed through the central brain, in response to the unopposed action of the lateral frontalis fibres.

The beginner is taught to look at a patient's face to get an understanding of where the important muscle complexes causing the dynamic rhytids are and how they work in each patient before treatment (Fig. 5.4).

Looking carefully at the patient's features will develop the art of SEEING. Several art colleges run courses on this for medical students (e.g. www.burrencollege.ie), and recent research has confirmed that art teaching is a powerful way to stimulate the powers of observation for ophthalmologists. The GOAL, as will be explained, is to be able to predict the treatment necessary to result in a satisfying resting tone, not necessarily a flaccid muscle complex. This is dealt with in more detail in Chapters 8 to 10.

Seeing Skills

Take photographs of your patient at the start of your consultation.

1. Examine bony contours of the face and socket for symmetry and note differences. In Fig. 5.5, note the differences in the socket dimensions, in the width of the face from the nose and

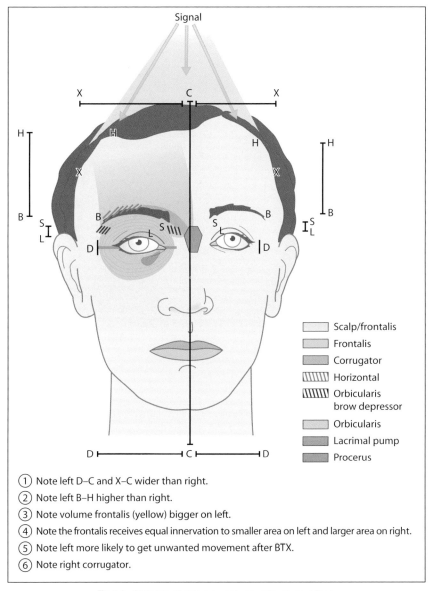

Legend:
- Scalp/frontalis
- Frontalis
- Corrugator
- Horizontal
- Orbicularis brow depressor
- Orbicularis
- Lacrimal pump
- Procerus

1. Note left D–C and X–C wider than right.
2. Note left B–H higher than right.
3. Note volume frontalis (yellow) bigger on left.
4. Note the frontalis receives equal innervation to smaller area on left and larger area on right.
5. Note left more likely to get unwanted movement after BTX.
6. Note right corrugator.

Fig. 5.4 Drawing of active muscle complexes on a face.

in the height of the forehead from brow to scalp. Differences between right and left measurements reflect different muscle bulk and different levels of innervation.

2. Manually examine the paired muscles of expression. Try to simulate the effect of BTX on particular muscle groups by depressing them manually while asking the patient to, for example, raise eyebrows. This will accentuate the diversion of signalling and indicate the best placement of injections to avoid peaking, etc. (Fig. 5.6).
3. Predict how a specific injection site will divert signalling to other muscles.

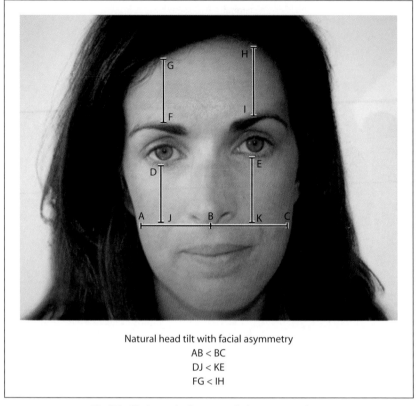

Natural head tilt with facial asymmetry
AB < BC
DJ < KE
FG < IH

Fig. 5.5　Photograph of asymmetric features on a face.

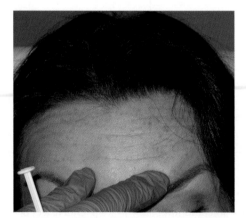

Fig. 5.6　Manually depressing the glabella while asking the patient to raise eyebrows.

4. Observe the anatomy of the patient's skull. Note in particular the frontal bossing of the forehead, note the line of the orbital rims, note the angle of the nasolacrimal fossa and note the lower lid to mouth distances.
5. Observe the difference in bulk between the same muscles on the opposite sides of the face. Allow for this when calculating the dose.

Discuss with your patients that they are different on each side, that BTX will have a different effect on each side and that you are going to modify your treatment to balance out the muscles. Remind them that you may need to see them for a touch up after the 'balancing' has happened. Let them know that you are training their facial muscles to soften where wrinkles form, while using other muscles to continue to maintain natural facial expression.

Control of Botulinum Toxin-A Placement

BTX-A can be injected to affect muscle position and tone depending on the patient's needs, as established by a practised visual examination as previously.

The degree of muscle contraction can be modified by injecting the BTX in four ways (Fig. 5.7):

1. Paralysis
   Placed intramuscularly.
2. Superficial paralysis with underlying active resting tone:
   the BTX-A is placed on the surface of the muscle.

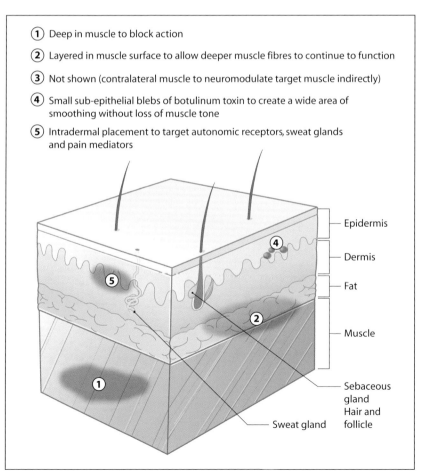

1. Deep in muscle to block action

2. Layered in muscle surface to allow deeper muscle fibres to continue to function

3. Not shown (contralateral muscle to neuromodulate target muscle indirectly)

4. Small sub-epithelial blebs of botulinum toxin to create a wide area of smoothing without loss of muscle tone

5. Intradermal placement to target autonomic receptors, sweat glands and pain mediators

Epidermis

Dermis

Fat

Muscle

Sebaceous gland
Hair and follicle

Sweat gland

Fig. 5.7 Drawing showing the levels of possible botulinum toxin placement through the skin.

3. BTX-A to the opposite muscle: for example, BTX-A to the brow depressors, allowing the frontalis to lift the brow unopposed (a BTX brow lift)
4. Placed in low doses over wider areas to 'neutralise' inadvertent signal from a treated muscle, with time allowing the resting tone to be maintained by the deeper layers

Placement can also be intradermal, affecting the sebaceous and sweat gland function, and probably the pain mediators.

Specific treatment choices will be discussed in Chapters 8 to 10.

USER TIP

It is prudent to invite new patients to return for observation at week 2–3, because at this point, it is possible to 'top-up' any unexpected overactivity of opposing muscles (e.g. causing brow 'peaking').

CHAPTER 6

The Art of Patient Selection and Short- and Long-Term Management

Some patients have a clear idea of their requirements and a good aesthetic sense. Others trust their doctors to advise them on 'what looks good'. They may come for treatment only because they were told to do so by their friends or their parents. If so, they may resent a treatment to which they are not fully committed.

The golden rule here is that if patients are not going to derive any perceivable pleasure from botulinum toxin, then their expenditure will not be properly rewarded. Their trust in their physician will be reduced, almost as if they had been 'sold' a dress in a shop that they did not really want—such shops are rarely revisited. It is important not to be influenced by such patients' demands. If the wrong decision is made by the physician and treatment is refused, then at least no harm is done. The botulinum treatment cannot be 'undone' 1 week later if the patient is unhappy with the outcome (even though the physician had already described the implications of treatment clearly). Above all, remember that no one NEEDS botulinum toxin for rejuvenation.

Patients frequently misunderstand the role of botulinum toxin and make an appointment to have it because they heard it advertised and want to 'lift' their face. It is a good idea to politely educate the patient as to how botulinum toxin actually works, and once they understand its effect on a muscle, inform them too about how wrinkles form.

How to Identify Suitable Patients

Listen to their presenting complaint and then, while still looking at the patient, decide quickly whether it can be treated with botulinum toxin or not.

Continue the consultation while carefully assessing the patient's psychological suitability (more later).

If, on first impression, the patient seems suitable, spend time providing verbal and written information about the treatment (this can be done by a trained nurse).

Always examine patients closely—as described in the following chapters—and discuss the likely outcome of botulinum toxin injections with them.

Be sure that your patients understand what has been said fully before they sign the consent form.

Selection Process

The decision must be made, prior to treatment, as to whether botulinum toxin can eliminate rhytids, reduce them and prevent further rhytids or whether another type of treatment is necessary. Consider whether patients are likely to look unusual after treatment (e.g. with peaked brows or tired appearance with heavy brows). Would they be better to avoid treatment altogether, to have gradual treatment over a few weeks or to have a different treatment?

TABLE 6.1 ■ Signs to Be Observed Quickly Before a Full Consultation Takes Place

Consider the following:	Look for:
General skin condition	Sun damage, pigment spots, poor tone.
Age	Cardiovascular status, skin perfusion, overall tone and skeletal structure.
Brow position	Examine lash/brow distance.
	How does it change with expression?
	Are the forehead wrinkles the result of 'holding' brows?
Crow's feet	At rest or in motion?
	Do they extend down towards the perioral lines when smiling?
Hooding	Is there a fold of skin at the corner of the eye that disappears when the patient lifts the brow?

The patient should have given an accurate age and history of smoking (Table 6.1) (although some do not!), and a full medical history reveals no obvious contraindications such as myasthenia gravis, pregnancy, etc. (see Chapter 7).

All new patients must be assessed physically and mentally. Written information about botulinum toxin should be provided at the time of consultation, and patients should have time to digest this before an opportunity is provided to ask the physician any relevant questions.

Initial Physical Assessment: Age and Skin Condition

With experience, it is possible to decide at a glance whether or not botulinum toxin will help a patient and what changes to the face may be expected as a result of the treatment (see Chapter 5 on neuromodulation). For example, a 29-year-old nonsmoker with crow's feet that wrinkle only when she is smiling will do very well (Fig. 6.1). Botulinum toxin will rid her of wrinkles completely. On the other hand, her sporty friend of the same age, who had not used adequate sun protection, may have wrinkles at rest with an early reduction in lower lid skin tone. Time must be spent explaining to her that she may possibly be disappointed with botulinum toxin—the injections might help to stop the clock and avoid new rhytids, but without alternative treatments (including sun protection, laser resurfacing, stopping smoking) she will continue to have her wrinkles.

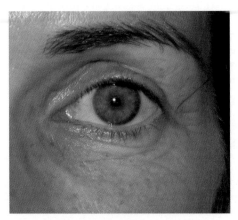

Fig. 6.1   Young nonsmoker with dynamic wrinkles only.

Expected botulinum toxin treatment outcomes may be addressed for short- and long-term management groups. Some patients just want a treatment for a special occasion; many patients resist the idea of long-term repeated injections. Other patients want a long-term maintenance plan in keeping with their personal health and self-care agendas.

SHORT TERM MANAGEMENT

Short-term treatment can be ideal for a special occasion and for many patients is their only affordable option. One treatment can quickly eliminate dynamic lines and soften the underlying static lines, but the effect almost always lasts only 12 weeks, particularly if the treated muscle is very strong. Suitability depends on age.

Crow's feet always return! It appears that the innate drive to smile, particularly as a muscle paired with perioral smile muscles for expression, is deeply embedded in our primal drive.

Patients may be reassured with photographs that regular botulinum toxin injections are not necessary to eliminate static rhytids and that these may be eliminated with CO_2 laser at any time.

Short-term botulinum toxin (e.g. one treatment lasting 12 weeks) is often indicated following CO_2 resurfacing to maintain a flat muscle as the skin recovers and builds up its collagen (Fig 6.2A and B, crow's feet pre- and post-CO_2 laser resurfacing).

Younger patients (<35 years old) do very well with 'one off' treatments. They respond quickly, and their underlying skin tone usually protects them from untoward thinning or sagging (Fig. 6.3A and B).

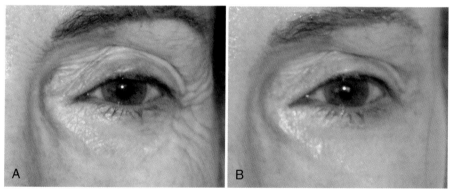

Fig. 6.2   Patient before **(A)** and after **(B)** botulinum toxin and CO_2 laser resurfacing for static wrinkles.

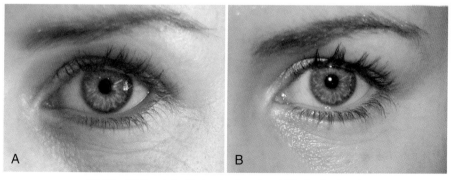

Fig. 6.3   **(A)** Crow's feet before treatment and **(B)** after treatment.

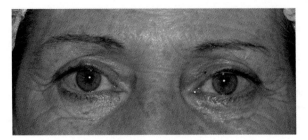

Fig. 6.4 Sun-damaged skin.

They can usually receive stronger concentrations of botulinum toxin to the full body of their muscles with maximum duration of effect.

Patients who present for the first treatment for their facial rhytids over the age of 45 years old tend to have limited knowledge of active skin care and ultraviolet light protection. Their rhytids are both dynamic and static. They often have premature brow sagging with blepharochalasis and ageing of their eyelid skin (Fig. 6.4).

These patients are strong neuromodulators of their muscle signalling. Any asymmetrical ageing, in keeping with any underlying basic asymmetry, is easy to spot. A careful examination will anticipate how they would look, should they select botulinum toxin treatment.

Older patients with sun-damaged loose skin, with reduced 'lift', are at a higher risk of the following undesirable outcomes to botulinum toxin injections:

- Dropping their brow resting tone, creating undesirable heavier brows and eyelid bags (Fig. 6.5).
- Developing vertical sagging of their lateral orbicularis, dropping their Sub orbicularis oculi fat (SOOF) suspension and therefore increasing and deepening their nasolabial folds (Fig 6.6).
- Reducing their lateral orbital rim volume, creating a 'thin' look, sometimes revealing vertical veins on the rim (Fig. 6.7A and B).
- Getting strong scalp overaction, 'crumpling' the superior third of their forehead when their frontalis is treated (Fig. 6.8A–C).

Such patients can do very well but could be advised to avoid having their first botulinum toxin treatment within 2 weeks of a major event, when the botulinum toxin would be fully effective. In the author's clinic, they are informed if it is obvious that they should have blepharoplasty first. Some can be successfully treated with a lower volume of botulinum toxin layered at the subcutaneous level, with a review for a top up at 3 weeks. It is often wise to recommend filler to the glabella for a short term fix (although it does last 9 to 12 months), rather than risk making the patient look worse with undesired loss of muscle tone. It is easier to 'train' the muscles gradually

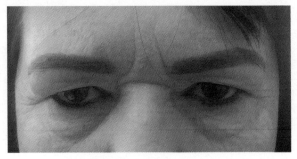

Fig. 6.5 Low, heavy brows.

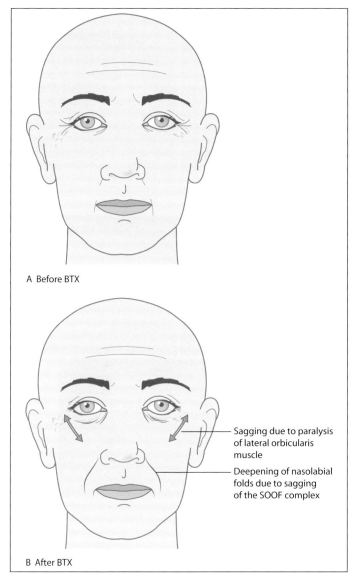

A Before BTX

B After BTX

Sagging due to paralysis
of lateral orbicularis
muscle

Deepening of nasolabial
folds due to sagging
of the SOOF complex

Fig. 6.6 Drawing of the lateral orbicularis rhytids before **(A)** and after treatment **(B)**, showing sagging of the sub orbicularis oculi fat *(SOOF)* after treatment, with deepening of the nasolabial folds.

with smaller volumes of subcutaneous botulinum toxin whilst keeping resting tone at the deeper layers of the support muscles.

LONG-TERM MANAGEMENT

A natural youthful look, the goal of the author's treatments, is one with plenty of facial expression, with a radiant complexion and with youthful natural facial volume balanced with the patient's own asymmetry. The patient must, above all, not look like he or she has been having any treatments.

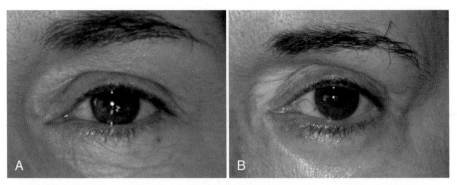

Fig. 6.7 **(A)** Before and **(B)** after botulinum toxin treatment: note thinning of lateral orbital rim.

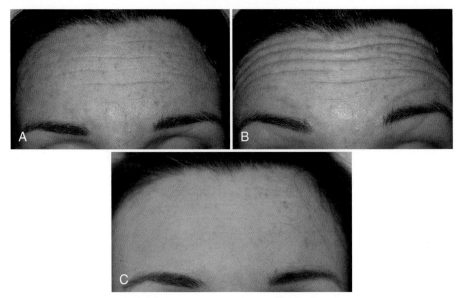

Fig. 6.8 **(A)** At rest before botulinum toxin, **(B)** moving forehead and scalp before botulinum toxin and **(C)** after botulinum toxin with movement.

Figs 6.9A, B and 6.10A, B demonstrate this in patients who featured in the first edition of this book in 2003 and now, in 2018, look almost the same.

USER TIP

The essence of good long-term management is to predict, anticipate and avoid untoward results!

Patients having long-term botulinum toxin maintenance should be told that botulinum toxin will eventually reduce muscle bulk and therefore facial volume. Advise them that they will have difference doses in different locations depending on their appearance at their first follow-up visit. These patients may come at various ages to 'start taking care' of their skin, etc.

In the author's experience, patients who started at a younger age frequently look better after 15 years of botulinum toxin treatments (Fig. 6.11A and B) compared with patients the same age who attend for the first time.

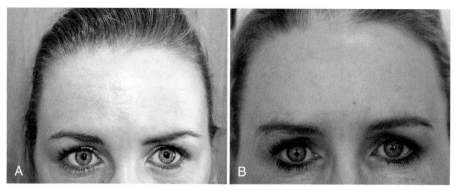

Fig. 6.9 **(A)** Before treatment and **(B)** 15 years later.

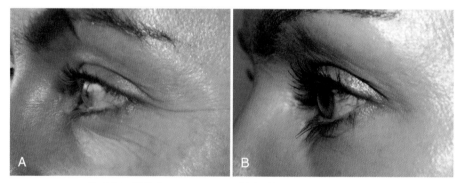

Fig. 6.10 **(A)** Before treatment and **(B)** in this edition, 15 years later.

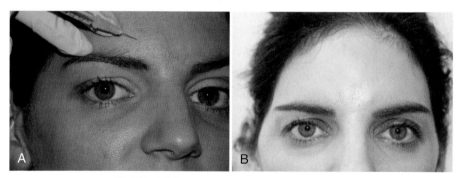

Fig. 6.11 **(A)** Forehead in 2003. **(B)** Forehead in 2018.

Patients who are older at presentation do especially well if they can first 'put the clock back' with CO_2 laser and blepharoplasties, then maintain movement and volume with filler and botulinum toxin.

If the patients have thin narrow lateral orbital rims, perhaps with prominent veins, they are sometimes advised to avoid botulinum toxin to their crow's feet, to maintain the more youthful muscle bulk. They may be suitable for fine hyaluronic acid filler or liquid fat to restore their rim volume. Static lines are treated with regular CO_2 laser and paraben-free Retin-A.

Long-term treatment is always planned with the effects of neuromodulation in mind. The patient learns, when observed before repeat treatments, that certain compensating muscles become too strong after a while and need to be weakened. For example, treatment of the glabellar complex for 'scowling' often diverts signalling to the lateral brow and when patients raise their brows, they manifest a 'peak' over the lateral aspect (Fig. 6.12). They will understand that the

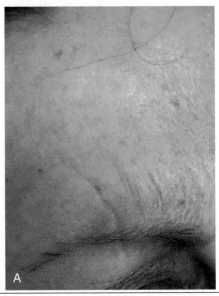

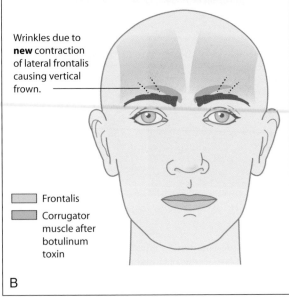

Wrinkles due to **new** contraction of lateral frontalis causing vertical frown.

Frontalis

Corrugator muscle after botulinum toxin

Fig. 6.12 **(A)** Lateral frontalis. **(B)** Diagram of lateral frontalis.

same muscles must not be continuously treated and that certain muscle complexes need to be allowed to recover and bulk up. This is to get the desired resting tone, natural brow position (without excess frontalis underaction) and a natural facial expression without static rhytids.

Long-term management is sometimes served best with multiple dilute injections layered on the anterior surface of the muscle, just beneath the dermis, accompanied by the occasional deeper intermuscular injection.

PSYCHOLOGICAL ASSESSMENT

The physician must develop a keen instinct when assessing patients for cosmetic botulinum toxin, in particular, the patient's psychological suitability and comprehension.

Aesthetic treatments, unlike medical ones, are not essential and can be refused at any stage. The initial consultation should identify patients who are poorly equipped psychologically to deal with changes in their appearance.

Every patient is entitled to follow-up consultations after he or she has received a treatment, regardless of the medical necessity of the visit. If a patient becomes distressed by the new shape of his or her eyebrows, it is important to be available to counsel and reassure him or her until the effect of the botulinum toxin has worn off. This is a rare occurrence but may even entail daily appointments for the first week, followed by weekly appointments for reassurance until the toxin has worn off.

GUIDELINES APPLICABLE TO ALL COSMETIC MEDICAL AND SURGICAL TREATMENTS

The first point of contact in a cosmetic practice may be the practice manager who books appointments and deals with patients' accounts. They too are trained to detect potentially challenging (unrealistic expectations, poor comprehension) patients. Patients frequently see an aesthetic nurse before their medical consultation. An experienced practice nurse can cancel a treatment plan for an unsuitable patient. The patients who eventually see the physician are usually ideal for treatment, but some are still deemed unsuitable at the time of consultation because of unachievable expectations or, more frequently, lack of psychological reserves to deal with a risk at that particular moment in time. Such patients may have their first treatment postponed and be given an appointment for review. A typical reason for postponement would be a recent bereavement.

There are obvious reasons for refusing certain patients even though they are physically suitable for botulinum toxin, but more subtle ones should also be considered.

The decision not to treat is always based on the possibility that the patient will not be happy with what the treatment will do—even if they think they will!

Ask yourself, before every new treatment, will this make this patient happy?

If not, why not?

SOME REASONS FOR POOR PATIENT SATISFACTION DESPITE A GOOD RESULT

Poor Comprehension

Patients who cannot understand risks or side effects despite repeated explanations often reveal themselves only after the first treatment, by telephoning the next day to say that it 'hasn't worked', or 14 weeks later to complain that the 'wrinkles have returned' despite advice about the time of onset and duration.

It is important for a clinician to understand that people have different ways of processing information. Most patients fall in to one of three, or a combination of three, categories: auditory understanders, visual understanders or tactile understanders.

A 'visual understander' grasps information quickly from pictures (e.g. pretreatment and post-treatment photographs), and they may not often 'hear' what is being said whilst taking in the image; an auditory understander 'hears' what is being said but quickly becomes saturated if shown more than one or two images; and a tactile understander has their information reinforced with processes, such a leafing through a brochure or filling out a form after learning of risks. It is the responsibility of the practitioner to provide enough information so as not to be misunderstood.

Unreasonable Expectations

Patients with unreasonable expectations often argue with the physician. For example, if shown how the brows might peak if their glabella alone is treated, they might disagree and continue to request the glabella treatment on its own. These patients also often reveal poor comprehension and deserve the extra time needed to allow them to fully understand what would be possible with their treatment.

Care must be taken to document in detail all consultations, with written information, photography and a good signed consent form. Certain patients may not remember ever being given information and have been known to inadvertently misrepresent medical advice.

The close friends of patients or their siblings can also have unreasonable expectations. One sibling, with a family resemblance, may marvel at the other's result and expect the same cosmetic result. It can be hard to point out that their sibling is a natural beauty with symmetrical features and good skin tone, whereas they, although rather alike, have lower heavier brows with asymmetrical frontalis action and sun-damaged skin!

Some patients are referred by other patients, expecting the same result as their friend. Care must be taken to explain the expected differences in results, while never referring to their friend or acknowledging that their friend really is a patient.

Depression

Recent research shows that botulinum toxin may actually reverse depression, by alteration of central neurotransmitter levels.

Depression is greatly underdiagnosed. Both reactive and endogenous types are relative contraindications to treatment. A depressed patient may speak slowly and seem 'flat' during the consultation. They may have suffered a recent bereavement, separation or divorce. Those who experience such life crises often review themselves. They notice their appearance, decide that they have 'let themselves go' and fix up a botulinum toxin appointment. Some become tearful during the consultation.

There are two good reasons for hesitating to administer rejuvenating botulinum toxin treatment to depressed patients. The first is the risk associated with every procedure; an unusual complication could deepen their depression. The other is that many patients, even mildly depressed ones, have poor powers of concentration, so they find it hard to assimilate medical advice.

The subject of their depression may be gently broached. Cosmetic treatment options may be discussed but perhaps accompanied with a suggestion to postpone the treatment until they are better. Psychological and medical counselling may be recommended, perhaps with a referral to their general practitioner for a psychiatric referral. Time is well spent discussing the way the body behaves with depression and the forms of treatment available. These patients usually return when they are better and are often suitable then for cosmetic procedures.

It is true that some depressed patients do cheer up when botulinum toxin eliminates their frown, but care should be taken about the timing of such treatments. Above all, they must be deemed healthy enough to provide informed consent.

Dysmorphophobia

This is rare but seen at every cosmetic clinic. It has various degrees of severity, and patients require a psychiatric referral—if they will agree to one. Avoid treating such patients without a report from their psychiatrist.

An example of a dysmorphophobic patient is one who came to the author for the management of an eyelid 'wrinkle'. There simply was no wrinkle where she pointed. In another, the normal lower lid morgagnian crease (between the pretarsal and tarsal orbicularis) was the offending wrinkle.

Such patients often refuse to look in the mirror during the consultation and almost always become distressed if attempts are made to photograph them. It is useful to remember that even though the defect identified by the patient is not apparent to the objective viewer, the patient may continue to view it as a problem whether it is treated or not. Some patients will have received numerous cosmetic treatments elsewhere at enormous expense. The ethics of this are debatable.

USER TIP

Avoid joint consultations (i.e. seeing two friends at the same time). Welcome a 'second ear' if necessary and let a friend sit in, but it is difficult to assess a patient's mental suitability for a procedure when speaking to two people at once.

CHAPTER 7

Contraindications and Complications

The right way to select patients for treatment with botulinum toxin (BTX) is described in detail in Chapter 6, and some well-established contraindications must always be kept in mind.

Absolute Contraindications

Anything that interferes with the predicted response to BTX, which inhibits the release of acetylcholine at the neuromuscular synapse (Fig. 7.1).

a. *Drugs and disorders which also reduce acetylcholine at the motor end plate, amplifying the action of BTX:*
- Eaton-Lambert antibodies. Note a history of cancer, metastases and general lack of well-being which may suggest a diagnosis of Eaton-Lambert syndrome (see 'Neuromuscular Disorders').
- Aminoglycosides (gentamycin, streptomycin, kanamycin) act on the presynaptic neurone.

b. *Drugs and disorders which alter the response of the motor end plate, amplifying the action of BTX:*
- Myasthenia gravis alters and reduces the acetylcholine receptors on the motor end plate (see section on 'Neuromuscular Disorders').
- Medication with succinylcholine (an agonist blocker) produces a prolonged depolarisation with reduced contraction.
- Tubocurare, pancuronium and gallamine are antagonist blockers that compete with acetylcholine for end-plate receptor sites.
- D-penicillamine can produce myasthenia gravis–type antibodies.

Drugs which reduce the action of BTX
The antimalarials chloroquine and hydroxychloroquine, and the immunosuppressant cyclosporin, can reduce the action of BTX.

Neuromuscular disorders
It is of paramount importance to avoid BTX in patients with neuromuscular disorders. Many such disorders are inherited and so a thorough family history must be taken with this point in mind.

General and local anaesthesia
Administering BTX at the time of general or local anaesthesia gives less predictable results. Avoid injecting BTX to the eye zone in patients who have had local anaesthesia for blepharoplasty.

Also avoid giving BTX in the postoperative phase where there is local oedema, to reduce the risk of distal diffusion and, for example, perioral palsy.

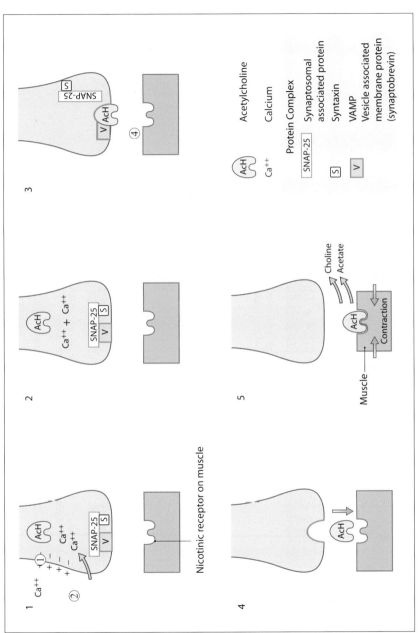

Fig. 7.1 Normal cholinergic transmission and action of botulinum toxin (BTX) at the neuromuscular junction: effects of drug and disease interactions (circled numbers). (1) Calcium channel blockers: aminoglycosides, cyclosporin; (2) tumour antigen antibodies block calcium channels (Lambert–Eaton syndrome); (3) block binding of BTX heavy chain to synaptogamin: chloroquine and hydroxychloroquine; (4) block nicotine receptor antibodies, e.g. myasthenia gravis, D-penicillamine; (5) postsynaptic acetylcholine antagonist: tubocurarine, galamine, pancuronium. Agonist blocker: succinylcholine. *Continued*

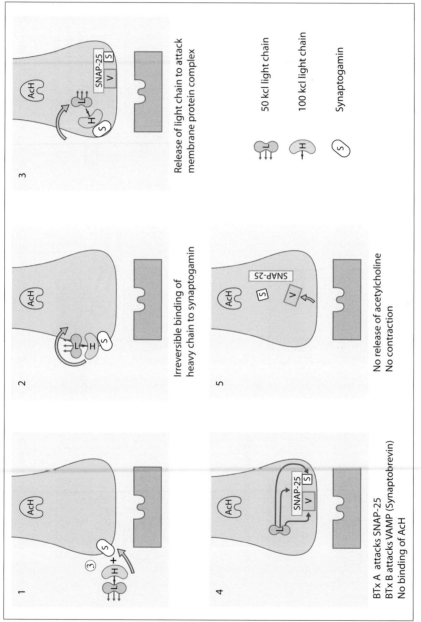

Fig. 7.1, cont'd

Contraindications:
Eaton-Lambert syndrome
Myasthenia gravis
Neuromuscular disorders (check family history).
Aminoglycosides (streptomycin, gentamycin, kanamycin)
Certain drugs used during anaesthesia (e.g. succinylcholine, tubocurare)
D-Penicillamine—used in rheumatoid arthritis
Chloroquine, hydroxychloroquine (antimalarials)
Cyclosporin (immunosuppressant)
Pregnancy
Infection

PREGNANCY AND BREASTFEEDING

The teratogenicity of BTX has not yet been established and so it is contraindicated in pregnancy and during breastfeeding. There are reports in the literature of dozens of women who inadvertently received BTX whilst unknowingly pregnant. One percent miscarried, and there appears to be no obvious association.

ALLERGY

A history of allergy to any ingredient in the formulation, including albumin. Reports of allergic reactions include local rashes. For noncosmetic patients requiring BTX (e.g. with cervical dystonia), IncaBTX-A (Xeomin), with its lower protein load, may prove a safe alternative but must be used judiciously.

> **USER TIP**
>
> Search the patient's history for any hint of muscle or nerve weakness that he or she may not be aware of. Enquire about episodes of intermittent drooping of the eyelid.

> **USER TIP**
>
> Take care to document that the patient has denied any contraindications.

Relative Contraindications

Many patients who come for BTX treatment for rhytids are self-referred. Their motivation is based either on a drive for self-improvement or a desire to 'have what their friend has had', that is a wrinkle-free forehead. Reserve judgement on their suitability for treatment until a careful assessment has been carried out. This is dealt with in detail in Chapter 6, and most of the side effects discussed can be avoided by rigorous patient selection. In addition, patients must be provided with detailed written information about the poisonous nature of BTX and the other risks associated with treatment.

If fully informed, most patients have reasonable expectations. Once in possession of all the facts, they are in a position to decide what risks to take and when. They may be happy to risk walking down the aisle with a camouflaged bruise or may prefer to postpone this risk until after their 'big day' and opt to keep their frown instead. If their treatment will be unpredictable (e.g. the treatment of a deep frown in a patient with moderate lash/brow distance and a moderate transient risk of immobile brows), then let them know about this. They can always change the date of their appointment to avoid it clashing with a big occasion.

USER TIP

Avoid treating patients who cannot fully understand the risks being discussed.

Table 7.1 lists the most frequent complaints encountered in the author's practice during more than 30 years of treatments with BTX for rhytids. During this time, the incidence of complaints has dropped dramatically, probably as a result of more rigorous patient selection and counselling, but also generalised public awareness.

Patient Complaints

COMPLAINT: IT DIDN'T WORK

Dysport and Azzalure usually start to work within 24 hours, but it is advisable to warn patients that results are not immediate and that they may notice nothing for up to 5 days.

It is possible to get a bad batch of toxin, causing a primary failure, albeit very rarely. Producers will replace a faulty vial immediately, free of charge, but rarely have to do so. Take care not to agitate the solution, and to follow storage guidelines carefully. The most likely cause for a failure of the toxin to work is inappropriate handling of it.

See the patients as soon as possible. Confirm that their treatment has not worked. It is wise to examine your files for other patients who received treatment from the same batch.

Offer to re-treat at no extra cost and reexamine within 2 weeks. If there is still no effect, advise the patients that they are resistant to the toxin and will have to pay for any further treatment using alternative toxins.

USER TIP

Advise patients to reattend with their complaint—but not earlier than 1 week and not later than 3 weeks.

TABLE 7.1 ■ **Patients' Complaints After Injections of Botulinum Toxin for Their Rhytids**

Complaint	Most Likely Cause
It didn't work!	BTX denatured.
It didn't last!	BTX too dilute or too old.
I'm still frowning!	Patients do not understand what you have told them about their low brows and the treatment of frown! (see Chapter 9)
Patient looks tired	BTX to forehead causes brow ptosis.
My eyes are swollen!	Due to protrusion of upper and lower lid orbital fat and skin from weight of flaccid brows and flaccid lower septum.
Hollow socket	BTX to inferolateral canthus in certain patients.
Peaked eyebrows	BTX over 75% of medial brow only.
Epiphora	BTX over lacrimal pump.
Severe bruising	BTX over branch of maxillary vein.
Unnaturally wide palpebral aperture	BTX to pretarsal orbicularis muscle.

BTX, Botulinum toxin.

COMPLAINT: IT DIDN'T LAST

Examine the patient if possible, but this complaint is usually made at a follow-up visit. Check the batch used and the other patients treated with it. The patient is usually right. The most likely cause will be excessive dilution of the BTX or denaturation by agitation or the wrong room temperature.

Reassure the patient. Consider reinjecting, but avoid doing so too frequently (i.e. within 12 weeks), to avoid the risk of stimulating antibody formation (see below). Use a different brand, a different strength or more sites, next time.

> **USER TIP**
>
> Patients who have suffered facial nerve paralysis (e.g. facial palsy) need smaller doses than often mandatory for effect because their facial muscles will be very sensitive to botulinum toxin following their denervation.

COMPLAINT: 'I'M STILL FROWNING'

Examine patients within 3 weeks but not before 10 days. This allows the toxin to take effect. Give more BTX if stray residual active fibres are genuinely visible. Spend more time on counselling if the result is what you have aimed for, that is some residual brow movement and lift in a moderate to low-browed patient.

Do not give more toxin to the lateral frontalis against your better judgment. A tired-looking patient will be far less happy than a partially frowning one.

COMPLAINT: THE PATIENT LOOKS TIRED

This is due to an unexpected lack of brow movement in a moderately low-browed person. It can also occur when BTX diffuses too far medially. The tonic orbicularis under the eyelid is loosened, allowing the infraorbital fat pad to protrude (see Fig. 6.6).

Spend time reassuring patients that the maximum effect is transient and that the extra muscles involved have received only the 'edge' of the treatment as the toxin diffused. This means that they will recover much sooner than the central muscles and that a tired look rarely lasts for more than 4 weeks. Increase brow movement with scalp aponeurosis exercises.

COMPLAINT: 'MY EYES ARE SWOLLEN'

A sudden onset of swelling and puffiness around the eyes, if pathological, is almost always due to allergy (associated with itch, hay fever, etc.) or infection (associated with erythema, pain, temperature). In the author's experience a local allergic reaction to BTX is uncommon, although this can occur in those who react to albumin. Care must be taken in the 60+ age group. Such patients have greatly reduced elasticity and tone. This results in sagging of the forehead skin (causing brows to drop) and sagging of the periocular skin (causing upper and lower lid bags).

Many patients use their frontalis muscle to suspend the sagging brows and upper lids. They hold their forehead muscle in a permanent frown, causing high arching brows and nice deep upper lids. Treatment of such a frown with BTX will automatically relax the frontalis, throwing their brows down and their lid skin onto their lashes. These patients may complain of droopy lids and 'swelling' over their eyes due to BTX, when in fact it is simply the skin sagging because the brow position has been lowered. Try to demonstrate this possibility to the patient by manually pressing their brows down. Avoid BTX unless blepharoplasty and/or brow lift has been performed.

Swollen eyes after BTX mean that the natural orbital fat and skin folds have protruded. Demonstrate this to the patient by asking them to look in a mirror with their head tilted upwards, a position that allows the fat to sink back into the sockets. Also lift the brows up actively with your hands while they watch the effect in the mirror. Reassure as described previously.

COMPLAINT: PEAKED EYEBROWS

This is dealt with in Chapter 9. Incomplete paralysis of the frontalis muscle is often chosen to achieve a natural effect. The aim is to retain some forehead movement while freezing the frown. The problem is that residual active frontalis fibres may sometimes, unpredictably, distort the shape of the brows. A symmetrical treatment may result in asymmetric brow peaking (Fig. 7.2). Some patients have naturally asymmetrical eyebrows: others experience contralateral overaction of untreated frontalis fibres as the opposite side fails to respond to stimulation. This is common in squint patients whose eye muscles work as part of a yoke mechanism. Contraction of the medial rectus on one side is associated with contraction of the contralateral lateral rectus. Under-activity of one muscle, for example the lateral rectus due to abducens palsy, will result in overactiv-ity of the opposite medial rectus (Herring's law).

Examine your patients carefully before starting treatment. Try to predict asymmetry (see Chapter 5). It is best to give an initial symmetrical treatment with a view to 'balancing' the effect within 2 weeks of the first treatment (Fig. 7.3A and B). Very little BTX is needed to achieve the correct effect (e.g. 0.025 mL [see dose box]) subcutaneously. Avoid using too much, because this can cause brow ptosis.

USER TIP

Individual facial muscles can be heavily interwoven or merge with neighbouring muscles, with plenty of anatomical variants.

COMPLAINT: A DROOPY EYELID

Ptosis is the term used for a droopy eyelid. The distance from the lower lid margin to the upper lid margin (the palpebral aperture) varies. Some patients have visible sclera below and above their limbus (edge of the cornea). This may occur naturally in myopic patients with naturally large eyes, in patients with thyroid eye disease or in those with unusually shallow orbits.

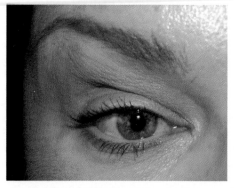

Fig. 7.2 Unnatural brow peaking following botulinum toxin to glabella in a patient with overactive lateral frontalis fibres.

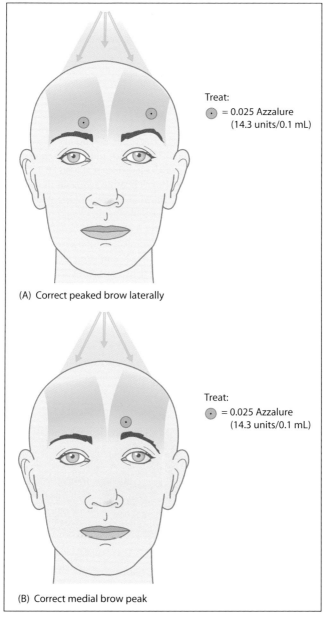

Fig. 7.3 Drawing to demonstrate correction of inadvertent lateral brow peaking. **(A)** suggests how to correct lateral brow peaking and **(B)** suggests how to correct medial brow peaking.

The eyelid is elevated by the levator palpebrae superioris muscle (normal range is 17 mm from looking down to looking up) and Muller muscle—a supratarsal collection of involuntary smooth muscle fibres. The voluntary levator muscle elevates the lid, while Muller muscle is responsible for fine tuning lid height and 'setting' it. Muller muscle is responsible for only 2 mm of lid height, and therefore paralysis (e.g. in Horner syndrome) causes only 2 mm of ptosis.

The upper eyelid margin of most patients rests 2 mm below the limbus and is symmetrical. Unilateral ptosis will often result in a raised eyelid on the other side, and likewise the illusion of ptosis can be created by unilateral lid retraction causing lowering of the opposite lid (Herring's law).

USER TIP

Always look for lid symmetry before giving botulinum toxin.

Congenital ptosis is relatively common (Fig. 7.4A and B) and age-related ptosis even more so. The latter is due to involutional weakening of the levator muscle attachments. It can be subtle at first (i.e. <1 mm) and is usually associated with elevation of the lid crease as the skin–muscle attachment separates from the original crease. Ptosis is often worse in the evening, and, in age-related ptosis, the eyelid will be lower than the normal lid on looking down (Fig. 7.5A and B). It is important to note that patients with levator aponeurosis disinsertion (age-related ptosis) usually raise their eyebrows to 'hold' the lid height. This can be a subtle change, and failure to detect it prior to BTX treatment will result in the unmasking of a preexisting ptosis.

There have been several reports of ptosis due to BTX, but some of these refer to brow ptosis, not to true ptosis. Brow ptosis will occur in any patient with an overactive frontalis muscle and involutional descent of the brows. It is not due to BTX to eyelid muscles, although brow ptosis can lead to an eyelid being pressed to a lower height by the simple effect of the weight of the brow on it. This can be identified by replacing the brows manually and observing the return of normal lid height.

True ptosis following BTX is due to inadvertent treatment of the levator palpebrae superioris muscle. Reported incidents occur if toxin diffuses through the orbital septum and usually last less than 2 weeks. The incidence is low and the author has seen only one case over years of experience with BTX, perhaps as a result of avoiding the levator muscle and never injecting medial to the

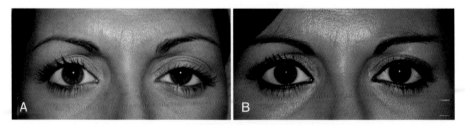

Fig. 7.4   Congenital ptosis: **(A)** before surgery and **(B)** after surgery.

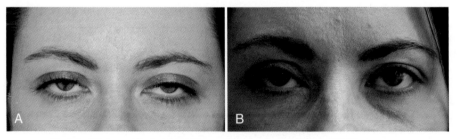

Fig. 7.5   **(A)** Age-related ptosis before anterior levator reinsertion. **(B)** After surgery.

lateral orbital rim. Unless experienced, practitioners should avoid injecting the corrugator muscle from the inferior aspect of the brow, particularly in patients with a low lash/brow distance.

Treatment of botulinum-induced ptosis is reassurance, reminding the patients that it will recover as the BTX wears off. Some recommend using Apraclonidine 5% (Iopidine) eye drops to stimulate the Muller muscle. This will result in a temporary elevation but only of 2 mm. Apraclonidine is an alpha-adrenergic stimulator used to reduce intraocular pressure and has several ocular side effects: its use in the treatment of transient ptosis occurring as a result of a cosmetic application of BTX is therefore questionable. The risks posed to the eye by use of apraclonidine must be balanced against the fact that the ptosis will undoubtedly recover when the botulinum wears off.

COMPLAINT: A WATERY EYE

Epiphora means a 'watery eye'. It is an unusual complaint but can either be due to paralysis of the lacrimal pump or to paralysis of the lower lid orbicularis.

Paralysis of the medial pretarsal orbicularis prevents the suction of tears into the lachrymal sac that normally occurs with blinking. It is often seen with Bell's palsy. It can be avoided by not injecting BTX medial to the mid-pupil line.

Another cause of epiphora is excessive laxity of the inferior pretarsal orbicularis.

The resting tone of the muscle is reduced and so the height of the lid drops. The increased palpebral aperture may undermine the normal tear film. The tear film break-up time may increase, and the ocular area exposed to the atmosphere may be too great for the volume of tears produced. This results in inadequate lubrication of the eye (a dry eye) BUT manifests itself as epiphora. When the eye is dry, the blink reflex causes the lid to pass over a dry surface, creating 'microscratches' on the cornea. This stimulates trigeminal nerve fibres and results in tears and a watery eye. Unfortunately, this reflex flow of tears is often not enough to cure the dry eye and may be accompanied by a gritty sensation. Remember that a reduction in the tear film, and mildly dry eyes, are common in menopausal women.

The treatment of epiphora due to pump inaction is to wait until the BTX wears off. The treatment of a dry eye is lubrication. Recommend over-the-counter preparations such as Tears Naturale, Artelac or Liquefilm. More viscous agents, such as Vidisic gel or gel tears, help if the patient is outdoors and at night. Lacrilube (petrolatum eye ointment) may be recommended in severe cases for use at night. If these measures fail, consider referral to an ophthalmologist for other types of management such as temporary lacrimal plugs.

OTHER COMPLAINTS IN TABLE 7.1

These are dealt with in Chapters 8 and 9. Experience in the art of BTX use will help to avoid them, and I rarely encounter them now. Having said that, Fig. 7.6 shows a recent patient who had BTX prior to lower lid blepharoplasty. Recommend a suitable camouflage cream.

Side Effects

The side effects of BTX are usually minimal: one of the deadliest poisons known to mankind is also one of the safest when used correctly.

USER TIP

Lessen the risk of developing resistance by avoiding booster injections and treatments less than 3 months apart. Use the smallest dose necessary.

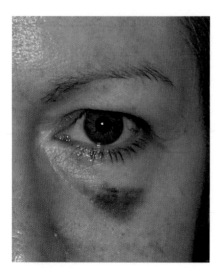

Fig. 7.6 Bruising following botulinum toxin injection to lateral canthus.

RESISTANCE

Most reported side effects follow the injection of toxin at high doses for the treatment of cervical dystonia and other large-muscle disorders. Antibody production has not been reported in patients receiving less than 50 units BOTOX. In one study, the production of immunoglobulin G auto-antibodies occurred in 4.3% of patients receiving BTX for torticollis. Those who have developed antibodies to type A should still respond to other serotypes. It is noteworthy that no resistance has been reported in patients receiving BTX for aesthetic reasons, but as patients receive higher doses to include neck rhytids, the risk of resistance must be kept in mind. Current advice is to avoid repeating injections within 3 months and to avoid booster injections

> **USER TIP**
>
> Botulinum toxin should be fixed inside intracellular tissues after 48 hours.

GENERAL

Patients have complained of generalised side effects, such as a 'flulike' illness and headache. Certain rare side effects such as generalised muscular weakness are believed to be due to the dissemination of BTX via the blood stream. There are electromyographic studies demonstrating contralateral effect for large doses for dystonia, presumably travelling retrogradely through the spinal cord. It is of paramount importance to avoid BTX in patients with neuromuscular disorders. BTX does not cross the blood-brain barrier.

Dysphagia can occur after the injection of BTX for cervical dystonia and is due to local diffusion from the injection site. The use of low-volume doses at high concentrations will limit this. Dysphagia has been reported following cosmetic use in the neck: neck weakness has also been reported. These symptoms usually subside after 2 to 3 weeks.

Bruising is an inevitable side effect of any intramuscular injection. Cutaneous vessels can be seen and avoided, but patients must accept the risk of ecchymoses from hidden vessels. Bruising in the lower lid can track down to the neck. Compress the injection site immediately after treatment and apply ice. Avoid injecting patients taking aspirin, nonsteroidal antiinflammatory preparations or *Ginkgo biloba*—a homeopathic inhibitor of platelet function—to reduce the risk.

CHAPTER 8

Management of Crow's Feet

'Crow's feet' are the wrinkles that form with age at the outer corners of the eyes. They are due to contraction of the orbicularis oculi muscles (Fig. 8.1). Their treatment with botulinum toxin is usually straightforward, but certain aspects must be considered carefully first.

The functions of the orbicularis oculi muscle are to close the eye, to drain the tear film and to create facial expressions. Contraction of this muscle can also drag on the lateral third of the eyebrow, contributing to drooping of the brow with age. In addition, the resting tension of the orbicularis oculi muscle can increase with age and character.

Many patients keep tension at the angle constant and so have pleasant 'smiling eyes'. This tension can be important to the appearance of the patient: it results in rhytids but also supports an ageing midface in some patients. It can also prevent the protrusion of age-related lower lid 'bags' (orbital fat) by supporting the orbital septum.

Injections of botulinum toxin will smooth out the rhytids and make the skin look younger, but patients may begin to look 'thin' around their eyes as they lose muscle bulk after repeated injections. They may also look 'drawn' or tired as their midface falls over the zygomatic arch. Such changes usually do not become apparent until several treatments have been undertaken. The loss of tension can reverse with time because the orbicularis muscle rarely atrophies permanently; this has been shown by the results of long-term botulinum toxin treatment of orbital blepharospasm.

This chapter covers the assessment and treatment of crow's feet. However, it is important to reexamine patients before every treatment and to make sure that they will still look well because of it. Make certain that the botulinum toxin can do for the patient what the patient expects.

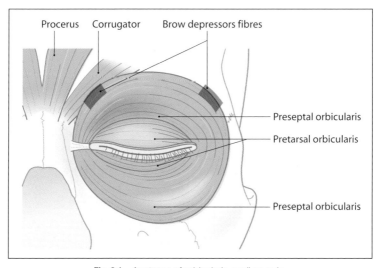

Fig. 8.1 Anatomy of orbicularis oculi muscle.

Patient Examination

Examine patients both from the front and the side.
Examine them at rest and when smiling.
Try to imagine what relaxation of their orbicularis muscle will do to their appearance.

What to Look for When Examining a Patient

- Examine the tone of the orbicularis oculi muscle and the position of rhytids. Are the wrinkles deep? Spread the skin gently between your fingers. Are they still very obvious? If they are, tell patients that they might not notice much effect from the treatment. Advise them about laser resurfacing and skin management. If the wrinkles are mild, advise patients that they might get a permanent effect with time and good skin care (Fig. 8.2A and B).
- Examine the facial skin and muscle tone by asking patients to smile while pressing lightly on the zygomatic arch with two fingers (Fig. 8.3A and B). This stops the orbicularis muscle from contracting and so simulates the paralysis of botulinum toxin.
- Patients with severe sun damage or poor skin tone (often older patients) will observe that, on smiling, the cheek and orbicularis oculi muscles elevate the facial skin and send it into folds around the lateral orbit. Show patients that this will also happen after botulinum toxin treatment to the crow's feet, otherwise they will think that the injections have not worked. It is often wisest not to treat such patients unless they have had surgical or laser correction of skin tone.
- The Mickey Mouse sign: occasionally, patients (especially men older than 50 with good skin tone) notice that smiling causes their wrinkles to 'bunch up' at the level of the zygoma after treatment of their crow's feet. This can create a curved wrinkle running from the lower orbital rim, out along the inferior border of the orbicularis oculi, over the zygomatic arch, to the top of the orbicularis oris (the Mickey Mouse smile). The periocular fibres have atrophied as planned, but the resting skin tone prevents elevation of the periocular skin and muscle on smiling. However, the excessive tone of the orbicularis oris, associated with thinning of lateral orbicularis oculi fibres, makes the smile appear much wider than the upper face. Take care with such patients.

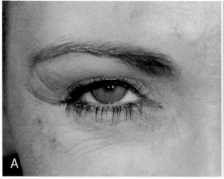 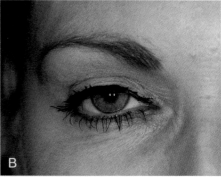

Fig. 8.2 One year before **(A)** and 1 year after **(B)** BOTOX to crow's feet.

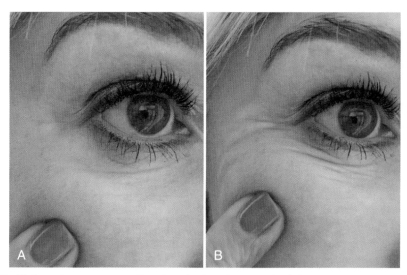

Fig. 8.3 **(A)** Press finger on zygomatic arch and ask patient to smile. This demonstrates the orbicularis muscle NOT contracting as if treated with BTX. **(B)** Push up skin from midface over zygoma. This demonstrates the effect of "smiling" on the midface and crows feet, independent of a BTX effect, in older skin.

- Examine the contour of the socket. Is it shallow, allowing anterior displacement of orbital fat and bags? Does the inferior orbital rim protrude? Is it recessed behind the level of the anterior surface of the cornea? This may also be assessed by the 'pencil test'. Ask the patient to hold a pencil vertically against the anterior cheekbone. If this passes in front of the cornea (Fig. 8.4A), then the patient has good lower lid skeletal support. If the pencil reaches only the lash margin (see Fig. 8.4B), before it would penetrate the globe, then the patient is at risk of developing sagging of the lower lid and widening of the palpebral aperture if botulinum toxin is injected for pretarsal orbicularis wrinkles.
- Examine the height and width of the zygomatic arch. Does the orbicularis muscle sag between the cheekbone and the eye? Will this area develop a hollow appearance if the muscle becomes

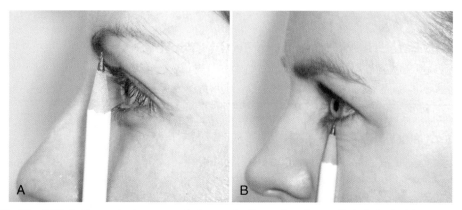

Fig. 8.4 **(A)** Typical bone structure means that a pencil will pass from the maxilla to in front of the cornea. **(B)** Some patients have a maxilla which receded from the inferior orbital rim. A pencil will pass from the maxilla through the eye. This means that inferoorbital contents (muscle and fat) are prone to bulging in front of the orbital rim, creating 'bags'.

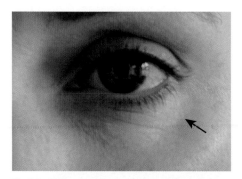

Fig. 8.5 Hollowing after botulinum toxin treatment. Avoid giving botulinum toxin on or medial to the infraorbital zygoma in a patient with high, broad cheekbones. This would cause atrophy of overlying orbicularis and subsequent hollowing. Note hollowing *(arrow)*.

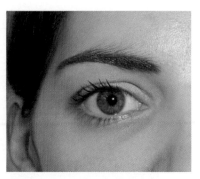

Fig. 8.6 Large eyes, wide, high cheekbone: Botulinum toxin close to the lower lid will weaken elevation of the lower lid and may increase the lateral palpebral fissure, creating a flat lateral lid instead of being angled above the height of the medial canthus.

thinner? Such a hollowing can be unattractive if accentuated (Fig. 8.5). Discuss this and inject more laterally to avoid diffusion to the 'hollow'.

- Take special care over patients with large eyes and wide, high cheekbones (e.g. Fig. 8.6). They are also, because of their large eyes, at high risk of sagging of the lower lid. The lower lid normally elevates with smiling as the palpebral aperture narrows and the orbicularis oculi contracts. Botulinum toxin will allow a more wide-eyed smile. This is often attractive, but never when the lateral corner of the lid falls below the medial, creating a pseudo lateral canthus inversus.

- Look for a weak orbital septum or protruding orbital fat pads. Ask patients to put their chin *down* and then to look up into the mirror—this will accentuate lower orbital fat pads. If fat protrudes, DO NOT treat the skin under the eyelid, because the subsequent loss of tone will cause temporary deterioration of the bags. These patients should have lower lid blepharoplasty and understand that only the wrinkles at the sides of their eyes will benefit from botulinum toxin.

Side Effects of Botulinum Toxin Treatment for Crow's Feet

These may occur if the injections are placed in the wrong part of the muscle, given at the wrong dose or given with unrealistic expectations. They are listed in Table 8.1.

TEAR FILM

Botulinum toxin to the eye zone can affect the tear film in two ways: the need for tear film may increase and the drainage of tears may be reduced.

Increased Need for Tear Film

Weakening of the pretarsal orbicularis widens the palpebral aperture. This may aggravate an already compromised tear film by increasing the area requiring lubrication and by reducing the rate of reflex blinking. Such patients may complain of a dry gritty feeling or, more likely, of watery

TABLE 8.1 ■ Side Effects of Botulinum Toxin Injections into the Orbicularis Oculi for Crow's Feet

Problem	Cause	Management
Thinning of muscle over zygoma	Injection in a patient with high, broad cheekbones	Inject more inferolaterally, below the zygomatic arch
Failure of lower lid to ascend with smile	Diffusion of botulinum toxin to pretarsal orbicularis	If looks well, repeat! If not, inject more laterally next time
Watery eye (epiphora)	Diffusion of botulinum toxin towards lacrimal pump preventing tear drainage	Avoid pretarsal orbicularis medial to midpupillary line
Hooding	Wrinkle due to sagging skin and not orbicularis contraction	*Counsel patient* carefully. Recommend brow lift surgery or cheat with hyaluronic acid
Large fold of wrinkles below zygoma (Mickey Mouse sign)	Patient has good result but poor skin tone, causing wrinkling of lower face only with smile	Discuss carefully
Patient may benefit from full face resurfacing or facelift. Botulinum toxin may be contraindicated otherwise

eyes. This is because drying of the eye causes the eyelid to scrape over the cornea and sclera, creating micro-epithelial defects and a sensation of grittiness. The resulting corneal stimulation provokes involuntary epiphora and a watery eye.

These patients should increase their artificial lubricants or lubricate occasionally with a gel substitute until the botulinum toxin wears off. Many lubricants are available without prescription, and the trick is to use them frequently initially, then to wean them off according to symptoms.

Reduction of Drainage of Tears

Botulinum toxin can be injected into the pretarsal orbicularis to reduce a hypertrophic orbicularis muscle and early 'bagging' (Fig. 8.7). However, it should never be injected close enough to diffuse towards the lower lid punctum. This would paralyse the lacrimal pump, causing a watery eye—unless, luckily, the patient was already suffering from a dry eye.

The lacrimal pump (Fig. 8.8) comprises fibres from the orbicularis that insert onto the vertical portion of the canaliculus and the lacrimal sac. Blinking contracts these fibres and dilates the canaliculus and sac. This creates a negative pressure drawing the tears along the lower lid margin into the lacrimal sac. Paralysis of the lacrimal pump occurs naturally in patients with facial nerve

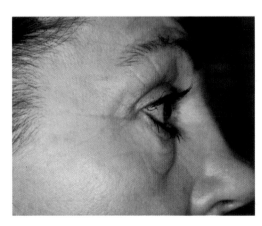

Fig. 8.7 Hypertrophic orbicularis muscle.

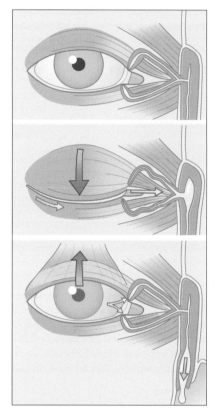

Fig. 8.8   Lacrimal pump diagram.

palsy. Treatment, if indicated, is by means of a glass tube (Lester Jones tube) inserted from the medial canthus to the nasal cavity.

Temporary paralysis of the lacrimal pump by botulinum toxin can be avoided by staying lateral to the midpupillary line and by using low doses of high concentrations. This treatment is not recommended for the novice practitioner.

LOWER LID BAGS (DERMATOCHALASIS AND/OR ORBITAL FAT)

Avoid injecting botulinum toxin medial to the outer orbital rim in patients with excessive lower lid skin and fat (Fig. 8.9), because this will cause sagging of the orbicularis muscle with protrusion of the inferior orbital fat. Remember, too, that botulinum toxin will diffuse to different degrees in different patients.

In the author's experience, an exception to the rule was a female smoker in her mid-40s with marked solar elastosis. She had botulinum toxin inferolateral to her orbital rim. She developed temporary heavy bags under both eyes as the toxin diffused towards the pretarsal orbicularis bilaterally. Fortunately, she received only the 'tail end' of the diffused toxin here and the effect wore off after a few weeks, long before the rhytids returned. It is very unusual for that level of diffusion to occur, and her poor skin quality was a contributory factor, but be warned! The same patient unfortunately refused to allow publication of her photographs.

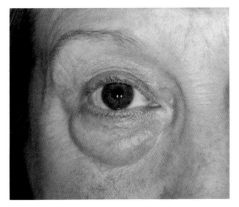

Fig. 8.9 Lower lid 'bags'.

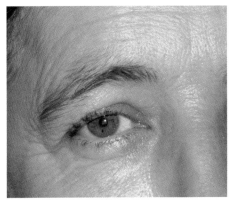

Fig. 8.10 Eyebrow ptosis.

Discuss blepharoplasty with such patients, and demonstrate what they can expect from botulinum toxin alone.

HOODING

Some crow's feet will persist despite botulinum toxin. These include the skin folds at the outer corners of the lids due either to brow ptosis or to sagging of the temporal frontalis muscle or both (Fig. 8.10). Discuss this with the patient and suggest correct surgical treatment of these wrinkles. Mention that 'cheating' with fine hyaluronic acid could also be effective (Chapter 11).

Method of Treatment

Crow's feet may be categorised and treated accordingly, as shown in Table 8.2.

Dose Box

BOTOX (BOTOX cosmetic): 2.5 mL dil to 100 units: 4 units = 0.1 mL
Xeomin: 2.5 mL dil to 100 units: 4 units = 0.1 mL
Azzalure 1 mL to 125 units (Speywood) giving 62.5 (Speywood) in 0.5 mL
Dysport 3.5 mL to 500 units (Speywood) giving 14.2 (Speywood) in 0.1 mL

TABLE 8.2 ▪ **Categories of Crow's Feet and Their Treatment**

Type of Crow's Feet	Management
Wrinkles in motion	Botulinum toxin
Fine lines at rest	Botulinum toxin, collagen stimulation
Deep wrinkles at rest	Botulinum toxin, laser resurfacing, ultherapy, radiofrequency
Deep wrinkles at rest with hooding	Botulinum toxin, laser resurfacing, hyaluronic acid, brow repositioning

Once the patient has been prepared, informed, examined and photographed and has consented, the recommended doses are as follows (shown on photographs); the reader is advised to visualise the centre point as the centre of a circle of diffusion, as taught in Chapter 4.

- Fig. 8.11: wrinkles in motion: 0.05 mL × 2 each side.
- Fig. 8.12: wrinkles in motion with lateral depression of brow: as previous with 0.025 mL lateral to point of contraction. Note the brow depressors are part of the orbicularis oculi fibres (Fig. 8.1).
- Fig. 8.13: wrinkles at rest extending over the zygomatic arch: as previous with 0.05 mL 1 cm inferolateral to lateral canthus.
- Fig. 8.14: high, wide cheekbone: 0.05 mL at outer canthus and 0.05 mL 0.5 cm below zygomatic arch.
- Fig. 8.15: treatment of crow's feet in older thinner skin: add in several shallow small doses ('bubbles') of less than 0.0125 mL by lifting the tip of the needle to raise a bubble/bleb. These should be placed where the wrinkles are shown to extend to as the patients smiles, over the zygomatic arch and towards the preauricular area.

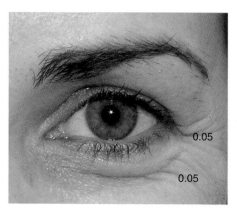

Fig. 8.11 Injection sites and dose for a young patient with wrinkles in motion.

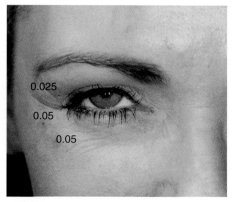

Fig. 8.12 Injection sites for wrinkles in motion and at rest with wrinkles below lateral brow.

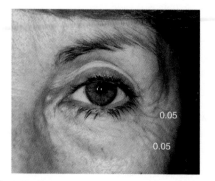

Fig. 8.13 Deep wrinkles at rest extending over zygomatic arch.

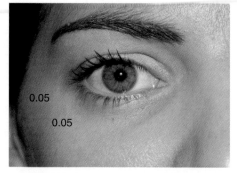

Fig. 8.14 Treatment of high, wide cheekbones.

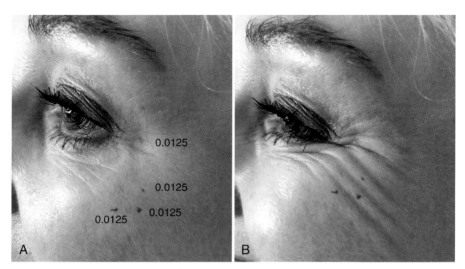

Fig. 8.15 Treatment of older skin with sub cutaneous microdoses over the zygomatic arch. **(A)** at rest and **(B)** smiling before treatment.

CHAPTER 9

Management of Forehead Wrinkles

Botulinum toxin is widely known to be an excellent treatment for smoothing out both vertical and horizontal forehead lines. Patients often ask for it to be used to treat their vertical (glabellar) frown or their horizontal lines or put in a general request for improvement. It is important to find out at an early stage whether they are looking for total immobility of the forehead (this is often not possible—as explained below) or simply for a natural-looking effect with some residual forehead expression and greatly reduced wrinkles.

Forehead wrinkles are due to a combination of genetic and environmental factors, especially damage ultraviolet light. The contributions of both must be analysed when patients attend for treatment. Make sure too that they do not expect the ablation of furrows as this requires carbon dioxide laser resurfacing for maximum effect.

Older patients tend to develop deep forehead furrows from subconsciously lifting their upper lid skin and brows off the eyelids. Ptosis or blepharoplasty surgery is often accompanied by relaxation of the frontalis and elimination of such rhytids.

Botulinum toxin to the mid-forehead can lead to permanent atrophy of the muscle fibres, with an excellent long-lasting result. This usually occurs after five or six treatments at 14-week intervals. The glabellar muscles always seem to recover after treatment but can, with time, diminish in size and function. Most patients continue to return for glabellar and crow's feet treatment, with an annual 'top-up' to the mid-frontalis.

Treatment of the frontalis will inevitably affect the shape of the brow. This must be assessed carefully and discussed with the patient. The treatment of horizontal lines alone may avoid changes to the brow, but once the glabella has been treated, the frontalis must be balanced with the treatment.

Remember that the shape of the brow is subject to fashion. I prefer the current trend for a female brow to have a slight arch at the junction of the medial two thirds to the lateral third. More modern trends include a horizontal brow that elevates laterally. It is essential to avoid a 'Dr Spock' effect with a peak to the brow, usually achieved by the unopposed action of the frontalis on the mid-brow, and most likely to occur when the glabellar muscles are treated independently.

Tell your patients what to expect from botulinum toxin at this stage, and discuss how their foreheads might alter with age. Let them know that with regular treatments, they will begin to lose their "reactive" frowning, as the central signaling area in the brain diminishes in size in response to their Botulinum toxin treatments.

Select patients as described in Chapter 6, and take great care to avoid treating the forehead of a patient with the rare neuromuscular disorder known as chronic progressive external ophthalmoplegia (CPEO). Remember that such patients may not yet have been diagnosed. Examine the eyes and eyelids of every new patient for signs of asymmetry or abnormal muscle function. If in doubt, refer to an ophthalmologist for examination before any treatment is attempted.

Chronic Progressive External Ophthalmoplegia

CPEO is a rare neuromuscular disorder that causes total immobility of all the external ocular muscles and of the levator muscles of the eyelids. Patients eventually need an operation to attach their frontalis muscles to their eyelids (by a subcutaneous sling) so that they can open their eyes and see. The initial presentation is often a symmetrical ptosis with brow elevation.

Anatomy of Frown Muscles

An intimate knowledge of the anatomy of the forehead is essential for successful treatment. There will always be a few patients with variations on the normal anatomy, but the typical muscle attachments are shown in Fig. 9.1. In particular, note the following:
  - The frontalis muscle originates from the galea aponeurosis (near the hair line) and stretches to an insertion into the skin and the orbicularis oculi at the level of the eyebrows.
  - The frontalis does not cross the midline and is separated by a central muscle-free zone at the base of the nose (Figs 9.2 and 9.3). Movements of the galea aponeurosis unaccompanied by movement of the frontalis will cause wrinkling of the forehead skin, especially in patients who can voluntarily 'wiggle their ears' or 'move their scalp'.

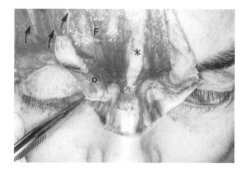

Fig. 9.1 Anatomy of the forehead. The vertical fibres of the frontalis muscle (F) insert into the skin and orbicularis oculi at the level of the eyebrow. The frontalis muscle, innervated by a branch of the seventh cranial nerve, originates from the galeal aponeurosis (G). The red arrow tip is inserted below the galea. The black arrow tip lies beneath the periosteum of the frontal bone. Note the sensory nerve (*), a branch of the supraorbital nerve coursing over the muscle. The frontalis muscle usually does not cross the midline. (From Zide, B. M., & Jelks, G. W. (1985). *Surgical anatomy of the orbit.* New York: Raven Press Books, Ltd. With permission of Barry Zide.)

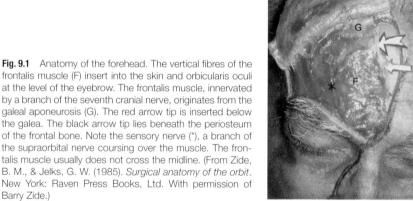

Fig. 9.2 Note that the frontalis fibres do not cross the midline. Note the paired frontalis muscles (F) with their central muscle-free zone (*). The supraorbital nerves are noted coursing upwards *(small arrows)*. The forceps grasp the anterior portion of the medial canthal tendon. Note the orbicularis oculi fibres (o), some of which originate from this tendon. (From Zide, B. M., & Jelks, G. W. (1985). *Surgical anatomy of the orbit.* New York: Raven Press Books, Ltd. With permission of Barry Zide.)

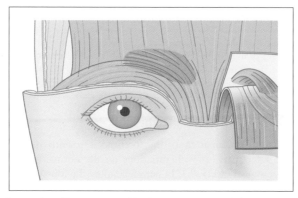

Fig. 9.3 The glabella complex. (From Zide, B. M., & Jelks, G. W. (1985). *Surgical anatomy of the orbit.* New York: Raven Press Books, Ltd. With permission of Barry Zide.)

- The bone at the base of the nose is covered by the procerus muscle (skin attachments only), blending into the corrugator muscle at the level of the eyebrows, and the medial fibres of the orbicularis oculi below the medial part of the brow.
- The corrugator muscle arises from the nasal process of the frontal bone. It is responsible for drawing the eyebrows together, creating the vertical glabellar rhytid. The corrugator lies deep to the frontalis, the procerus and the supraorbital nerves and arteries. It attaches to the skin above the medial aspect of the eyebrow.

The vertical fibres of the orbicularis oculi, which run superomedial to the medial canthal tendon, attach to the medial brow and are known as the depressor (corrugator) supercilii. The angular veins are embedded in this muscle.

Examination of Brow/Forehead Rhytids

General appraisal
Specific glabella (vertical frown) examination
Specific forehead (horizontal frown) examination

GENERAL APPRAISAL

Brows
Hairstyle
Ptosis
Dermatochalasis

First, examine your patient carefully and decide what botulinum toxin can do for his or her particular type of lines. Decide at this stage whether or not botulinum toxin treatment will eliminate the wrinkles. Will laser resurfacing be needed? Will the vertical lines also require a filler (Chapter 11)?

Eyebrows

Examine the eyebrows. Are they heavy or groomed? Some brows look as if they have descended because of their excessive growth of hair. Simple contouring of the brow with tweezers can give the illusion of a lift and instantly take years off the eyes (Fig. 9.4A and B). A visit to a reputable beautician may be recommended to acquire a professional shape, which the patient can easily maintain thereafter.

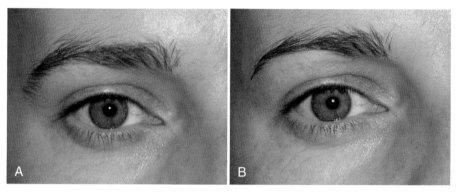

Fig. 9.4 (A) Before and (B) after eyebrow contouring.

Hairstyle

Discuss this with the patient. If a fringe (bangs) is being worn, will the effects of botulinum toxin be noticeable? Is the patient happy to have botulinum toxin to prevent further ageing of the forehead, regardless of whether or not it can be seen? Is the patient getting a receding hairline with widow's peaks? This can be ageing. Full forehead and scalp botulinum toxin treatment will lengthen the forehead further. They may be advised to modify their hairstyle to hide the receding areas. Has the patient seborrheic dermatitis, acne rosacea or psoriasis? In the author's experience, this usually disappears in the zones treated with botulinum toxin, to the delight of the patients. Inform them of this possible bonus.

Ptosis

Always examine the patient for signs of ptosis (a droopy eyelid). This is common in patients over 60 years old and is usually unilateral or asymmetrical. The levator aponeurosis, which opens the eyelid, and which is also responsible for the 'lid crease' by its superficial insertion into the orbicularis muscle and skin, slips up under the orbital rim (and eyebrow) with age or trauma, including eye rubbing. This causes a slight drooping of the eyelid that worsens on looking down and when the patient is tired (Fig. 9.5A and B). Patients then compensate by tensing the frontalis muscle,

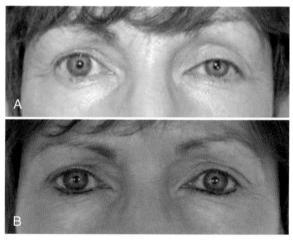

Fig. 9.5 (A) Before and (B) after left levator aponeurosis reinsertion. Note high lid crease and ptosis preoperatively.

developing high arched eyebrows, deep frontalis furrows and deep upper lids, which droop sleepily. The lid crease is often noticeably higher on the affected side (normal 7 to 10 millimeters, symmetrical).

In these patients, botulinum toxin to the frontalis muscle results in an immediately obvious ptosis (even though it was already present). Patients will also complain of the appearance of swollen upper lids as their brow descends. The ptosis is often asymmetrical, sometimes unilateral, and sometimes occurs in young people following trauma. It will be hard to convince these patients that the botulinum toxin did not cause the initial ptosis. Examine carefully before treating!

Basic Ptosis Examination

- Observe the patient in the primary position (looking straight ahead).
- Measure the palpebral aperture (P.A.)—the distance from the lower lash margin to the upper lash margin at the midpoint of the pupil.
- Place a finger over the patient's brow to stop it from moving.
- Ask the patient to look down. Place the zero point on a fine ruler over the upper lid lashes before immediately asking the patient to look up. Now measure the point on the ruler where the lash margin has risen to.
- The result is the levator muscle function (normal is 15 to 18 mms).

Dermatochalasis (Eyelid Bags)

The term dermatochalasis refers to age-related wrinkling and sagging of the skin over the eyelids. Examine carefully for brow elevation with overaction of the frontalis compensating for the 'heavy skin' and subconsciously lifting it off the lids (Fig. 9.6). Botulinum treatment to the frontalis may unmask the dermatochalasis and give the illusion of 'swelling' of the upper lid skin (Fig. 9.7A and B).

EXAMINATION OF THE GLABELLAR FROWN

The glabella is the area between the eyebrows. A deep rhytid, the glabellar crease, may occur in isolation (Fig. 9.8); with a parallel but usually shorter rhytid (Fig. 9.9); or with curved rhytids under the medial brows (Fig. 9.10). A vertical glabellar crease is usually associated with hypertrophy of the medial corrugator fibres.

Horizontal glabellar rhytids ('Bunny Lines') are due both to dynamic and static factors. The dynamic cause is contraction of the procerus muscle (there is no frontalis here). The static cause is sagging of the forehead skin and muscle with age, overhanging the base of the nose (Fig. 9.11).

The medial fibres of the frontalis elevate the brow but overlie the brow depressor and the corrugator. Treatment of the corrugator should avoid the brow elevator fibres.

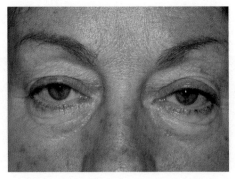

Fig. 9.6 High raised eyebrows with forehead wrinkles and upper eyelid bags, and 'bag' weight induced ptosis.

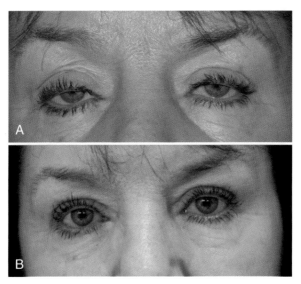

Fig. 9.7 **(A)** Before and **(B)** after upper eyelid surgery for dermatochalasis, unmasked by botulinum toxin to the forehead.

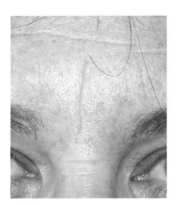

Fig. 9.8 Single vertical frown in a 40-year-old woman.

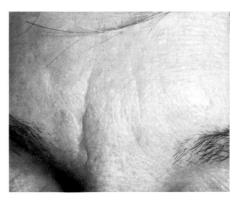

Fig. 9.9 Parallel vertical frown lines.

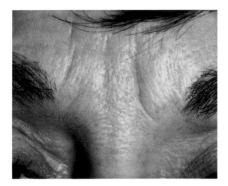

Fig. 9.10 Curved vertical frown lines.

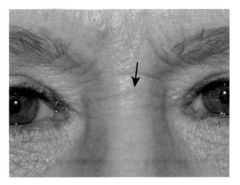

Fig. 9.11 Bunny line.

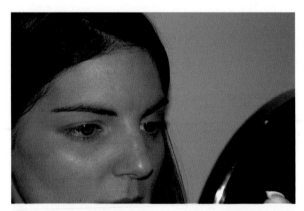

Fig. 9.12 Ask the patient to close both eyes (allowing eyebrows to drop), then to open eyes slowly while looking in a mirror. This demonstrates the probable resting position of the brows after botulinum toxin A to the frontalis muscle.

EXAMINATION OF THE HORIZONTAL FROWN

Examine the brows carefully. First, demonstrate the effect that botulinum toxin to the forehead would have if brow tone were to be weakened. To do this, ask the patient to close both eyes and then to open them very slowly while looking in the mirror. This may require repeated attempts, but show the result to the patient in the mirror (Fig. 9.12)

Examine the upper lid crease once this has been achieved. If the lid crease is unaltered by their resting brow, then the patient is suitable for full botulinum toxin treatment. If the lid crease has become full due to dermatochalasis or mild brow ptosis, recommend a limited botulinum toxin treatment to the upper forehead and advise the patient that some movement of the forehead will remain.

Brow Examination

1. Observe where the horizontal and vertical forehead rhytids lie. Are they due to excessive brow elevation? Is the patient holding an excess of upper lid skin off their lids? Explain to the patient that botulinum toxin may make them look too 'tired' or 'heavy lidded'. They will be open to a partial effect or surgical alternatives.
2. Tug on the skin below the brow to check for laxity. Does the brow droop at the sides? Tell patients that they might get a temporary elevation of the lateral brows after treatment (Fig. 9.13) but that this is not always repeatable as some frontalis fibres eventually atrophy.
3. Ask patients to elevate their brows. Are they symmetrical? (Most are not.) Point out any asymmetry.
4. When the brows are elevated, do they 'peak' at any point? Some patients have naturally pointed brows which, if unmasked with botulinum toxin, look unattractive (Fig. 9.14A and B). The currently fashionable arch lies at the junction of the medial two thirds and the outer third of the eyebrow—but fashions change.
5. Ask the patient to frown (Fig. 9.15A and B). Which fibres contract? Some patients actually elevate their medial brow by contracting the corrugator, raising the brow superomedially. Others tend to drag the brow down.
6. Decide whether or not the patient would benefit from an endoscopic brow lift or blepharoplasties (Fig. 9.16A and B). Discuss this with them and refer if necessary. Explain the

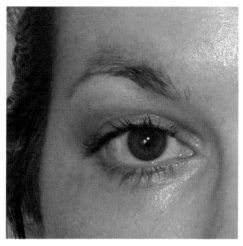

Fig. 9.13 Temporary elevation of lateral brow, creating a pleasing arch after Botox to the glabella. Note post-laser resurfacing erythema (10 days post-laser).

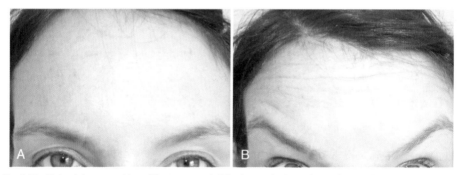

Fig. 9.14 Natural brow peaking: **(A)** at rest and **(B)** when asked to elevate brows, before receiving any botulinum toxin treatment.

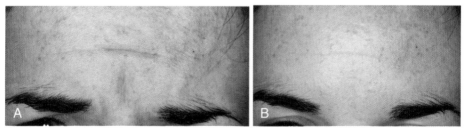

Fig. 9.15 **(A)** Before and **(B)** after Botox for frowning. Patient is trying to frown in **(B)**.

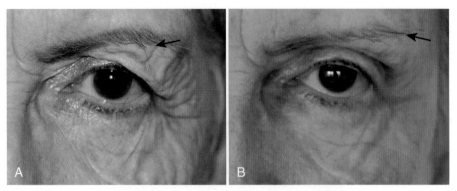

Fig. 9.16 **(A)** Before and **(B)** after endoscopic brow lift for brow ptosis. Note that the eyebrow in **(A)** has been 'drawn in' at a higher level than the real brow hairs, shown post operatively (arrow) in **(B)**.

improvements possible from botulinum toxin without surgery (use your hands to stabilise the medial brow, for example, while the patient raises the brow).

7. On the follow-up visit, before the next treatment, ask patients to place their fingers over their brow muscles and feel the contraction as they frown. They will often notice that the lateral fibres of the frontalis have strengthened, squeezing the corrugator toward the glabellar area. Some patients may tolerate botulinum toxin to this lateral area, but most will look tired, with total inaction of their frontalis if treated. Of significance is that these fibres can strengthen with successive glabellar treatments, 'pushing' in the frown again despite atrophied corrugators. The edge of a diffusion circle of treatment may be used to weaken these fibres.

Principles of Forehead Rhytid Treatment (See Fig. 9.26)

The mid-frontalis may eventually atrophy, requiring less treatment.
The glabellar complex rarely atrophies.
Treatment changes with time as the muscle response alters.
Untreated muscle can hypertrophy with time, for example the lateral frontalis.
Treatment depends on brow position and the presence or absence of blepharochalasis.
Avoid ptosis by not injecting beneath the superior orbital rim.
Avoid peaked brows by lightly treating the frontalis 2 cm above the possible peak.
Avoid intramuscular injections close to or in the brow.
Discuss brow movement at length with the patient.

Recommended Treatment of Forehead Wrinkles
(See Tables 3.4 and 3.5)

Dose Box

Botox: 2.5 mL to 100 units = 4 units per 0.1 mL
Xeomin: 2.5 mL to 100 units = 4 units per 0.1 mL
Dysport: 3.5 mL to 500 units = 14.3 units per 0.1 mL
Azzalure: 0.63 mL to 125 units = 10 units per 0.05 mL

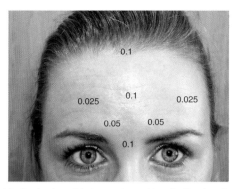

Fig. 9.17 Suggestion for glabellar treatment in inexperienced hands. Forehead complex and scalp must be balanced to avoid peaking.

The forehead is best treated as a single zone to achieve a balanced effect. Consider the optimal glabellar treatment and then treat the frontalis accordingly.

Basic Glabellar Treatment (Fig. 9.17)

Treatment of a glabellar rhytid:

The essence of treatment is to paralyse the contraction of the corrugator muscle while allowing acceptable brow movement WITHOUT descent of the medial brow or ascent of the lateral brow! The author rarely treats the glabella alone, because most patient examinations reveal probable diversion of signalling to the frontalis over a peaked brow. This is usually avoided by giving 0.025 mL to the point of peaking.

Visualise diffusion circles as in Fig. 9.26. Inject 0.05 mL to 0.1 mL, depending on muscle bulk, 1.5 to 3 cm above medial brow (line of medial canthus). ALWAYS aspirate first to avoid the supraorbital complex. Inject 0.1 mL at the base of nose below brow level (to diffuse across 3 cm to procerus and brow depressors). Note that the procerus often resembles a pentagon when contracted. Inject 0.025 mL 1 cm above the base of corrugator muscle, aiming not to depress the natural brow arch.

> **USER TIP**
>
> Use palpation to augment observation when assessing the location of maximum muscle contraction during frowning.

Advanced Glabellar Treatment

With experience and finesse, it is possible to inject smaller volumes of higher concentrations of botulinum toxin. Injections can then be placed below the brow, up towards the corrugator muscle and above the trochlear tendon towards the medial brow depressor fibres. Until then, inject allowing for a wider diffusion zone to avoid unwanted diffusion. Great caution must be taken not to enter a blood vessel in the very vascular area of the superomedial orbit. Inaccurate dosage may cause toxin to diffuse towards the levator muscle, causing ptosis, and toward the superior oblique muscle, causing diplopia. Outstanding results may be achieved with low volumes of high concentrations, with subtle elevation of the brows and smoothing of all furrows. However, this technique should be undertaken only by those completely familiar with anatomical variations in this area who are experienced enough to assess the degree of diffusion of the different concentrations accurately (Fig. 9.18A and B).

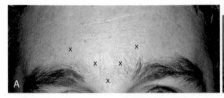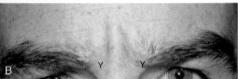

Fig. 9.18 Suggested injection sites *(X)* for optimal glabellar treatment in inexperienced hands. **(A)** Before and **(B)** after frowning. Site *Y* is at high concentration and low volume to avoid ptosis. Do not try unless comfortable with diffusion distances.

Important Considerations for Glabellar Treatment

Injecting botulinum toxin below the orbital rim greatly increases the risks of true ptosis (a droopy eyelid) due to diffusion of toxin towards the levator muscle of the lid.

The corrugator may be approached from below the medial brow by an expert, thereby avoiding the elevating frontalis fibres. Lower doses at higher concentrations are recommended—but only in experienced hands.

The supraorbital artery, vein and nerve lie on the corrugator muscle and must be avoided. Palpate the supraorbital notch (not always present) in the bone just medial to the medial brow. This is the line of the supraorbital complex (2.7 cm from midline).

The angular vein traverses the area below the medial brow, the site of the depressor supercilia.

Basic Frontalis Treatment

Examine the frontalis region by asking the patient to frown repeatedly, allowing identification of the strong points of the frontalis. Inject the bulk of the muscle adjacent to the rhytid. Inject 0.01 mL intramuscularly in the central zone as shown (Fig. 9.19) and then inject 0.05 mL to the other areas to give symmetry. An injection of 0.025 mL subcutaneously above the mid-lateral brow can soften rhytids whilst retaining frontalis action. On follow-up visits, inject 0.1 mL into the scalp aponeurosis to discourage hypertrophy and an overaction of aponeurotic fibres, which would result in excessive scalp movement relative to the atrophic frontalis muscle (Fig. 9.20).

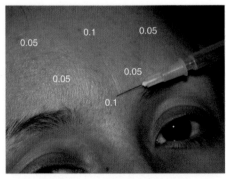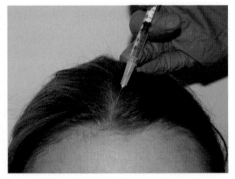

Fig. 9.19 Basic frontalis treatment.   **Fig. 9.20** Injection to scalp aponeurosis.

USER TIP

Tell the patient that the treatment sites will be different each time because the muscles will recover differently.

Different Types of Rhytids May Be Treated as Follows:

Fig. 9.21A: Simple forehead lines in motion, none at rest (20 to 30 years).

If the brows are firm, then treat the complete frontalis. Expect a semi-permanent effect within 2 years as the frontalis muscle atrophies.

Young patients with firm brow attachments are easy. Inject the glabellar area as shown in Fig. 9.18, along the line of the corrugator. Treat the frontalis as shown to prevent peaking of the brows. Injection sites are chosen to allow for diffusion of the toxin within 1 to 3 cm of the site. This allows treatment of the procerus medially, sometimes incorporating some overlying frontalis fibres with diffusion towards the brow depressor, counteracting brow depression medially at the most nasal aspect of the brow. Fig. 9.21B shows the same patient as in Fig. 9.21A, 15 years later!

Fig. 9.22: Simple forehead lines in motion, none at rest (20 to 30 years).

Short brow lash distance with slightly mobile brows. Avoid lateral frontalis and treat supero-lateral frontalis instead. Treat medial brow depressors.

Fig. 9.23: Forehead lines at rest and in motion.

Treat as above but classify rhytids. If severe, advise about CO_2 resurfacing.

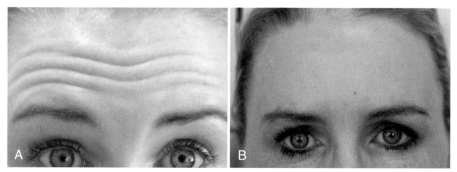

Fig. 9.21 **(A)** Before simple forehead lines in motion, none at rest (20 to 30 years), and **(B)** after treatment, 15 years later.

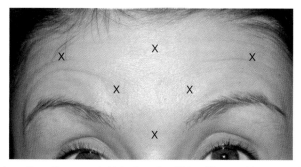

Fig. 9.22 Wrinkles in motion with suggested injection sites *(X)* in a 20-year-old woman with short lash-brow distance and mobile brows.

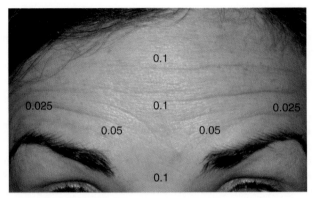

Fig. 9.23 Suggested injection sites with suggested doses in a patient over 40 with high arched brows and wrinkled forehead, note the sites are NOT symmetrical, in keeping with the asymmetrical frontalis mass.

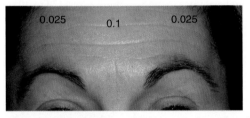

Fig. 9.24 Suggested doses and injection sites in a patient over 35 with high arched brows and wrinkled forehead. Retain brow height, if desired, by avoiding botulinum toxin to brow area (i.e. lower half of forehead).

Fig. 9.24: High arched brows with furrowed horizontal lines in patient over 35.

Take great care. This patient is typical of those who can become extremely distressed if they lose the deep appearance of their upper eyelids as the frontalis becomes paralysed with botulinum toxin. The heavy brow can sometimes weigh upon the upper lid simulating ptosis; but when the brow is gently lifted by the examiner's finger, the lid will return to its normal position.

Discuss surgical correction at length (Chapter 11). Consider botulinum toxin treatment to the upper rhytids, retaining the elevating action of the lower frontalis fibres. Offer filler to the glabellar crease and the fine lines over the lateral brow.

Fig. 9.25: The male forehead.

The male brow tends to be horizontal with a short lash brow distance. The muscles may be bulkier than those of the female forehead and sometimes need greater doses. Treatment of the glabellar area *per se* can lead to a feminising arch and must be avoided unless requested. The male forehead is also prone to a receding hairline. Such patients may require extensive volumes of botulinum toxin to treat the occipito-frontal portion of the frontalis; otherwise, they will return with frontal furrows.

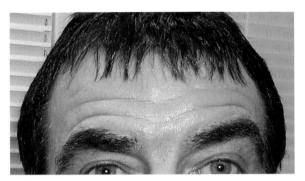

Fig. 9.25 Typical heavy male forehead.

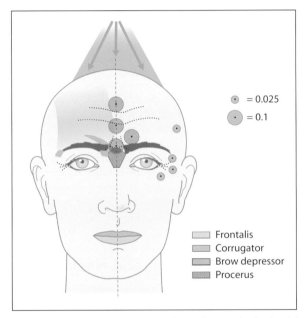

Fig. 9.26 Low heavy brows. Note the signal to raise brows is equal across the forehead *(green rays overhead)* before treatment. The pink circles of diffusion are used to overlap the corrugator *(blue)* and the procerus *(grey pentagon)* and the brow depressors *(pale green stripes)*. Note the space between the circles *(pale green stripes on forehead)* are left to allow lift and shape.

CHAPTER 10

Treatment of the Perioral Region, the Neck and Scars

Dose Box (see Tables 3.4 and 3.5)

BOTOX 2.5 mL to 100 units, 4 units in 0.1 mL
Xeomin 2.5 mL to 100 units, 4 units in 0.1 mL
Dysport 3.5 mL to 500 Speywood units, 14.3 units in 0.1 mL
Azzalure 0.63 mL to 125 Speywood units, 10 units in 0.05 mL

A good knowledge of the anatomy of the perioral region is essential before undertaking botulinum toxin treatment. The orbicularis oris responds well to botulinum toxin, but great care must be taken to limit diffusion into the surrounding muscles (Fig. 10.1). This can be achieved by using a higher concentration of the toxin, at a smaller dose. Treatment of the wrong muscle fibres can lead to dribbling, difficulty in drinking water, slurred speech and asymmetrical smiling.

Patients with facial hemispasm frequently require botulinum toxin to a focus of spasm over the elevator of the lip. This leads to a depression of the corner of the mouth and drooling of saliva (Fig. 10.2). But patients would usually rather have an embarrassing dribble than an uncomfortable spasm and twitching of the side of their face. However, this complication MUST be avoided in a cosmetic practice.

Ageing of the Perioral Region and Neck

Ablating wrinkles does not always make a patient look younger. When considering rejuvenation of this area, examine the overall tone of the musculocutaneous complex. Also examine the skeletal support, the dentition and the shape of the nose.

Research has confirmed that ageing causes an anteropostero recession of the facial bones, which contributes to sagging. The distance from the nose to the vermilion border increases with time. The vermilion border itself shrinks, and the lips lose volume and tend to turn downwards instead of up and out.

The lip depressors and elevators induce wrinkles at the corners of the mouth and 'marionette lines'. The mentalis muscle encourages the tip of the chin to turn upwards, creating the mental fold and sometimes a 'pointed' chin. Recession of the jaw will accentuate the wrinkles, from the corner of the mouth to the chin.

The platysma muscle will eventually draw the sides of the mouth towards the jaw, and this, along with facial sagging, creates jowls. Increased resting tone of the platysma creates vertical bands (turkey neck) along the line of action and 'venus rings', that is horizontal banding, perpendicular to the line of action.

The tip of the nose becomes pulled down with time (pointed nose) and the descent of the midface, coupled with recession of the facial bones, deepens the nasolabial folds.

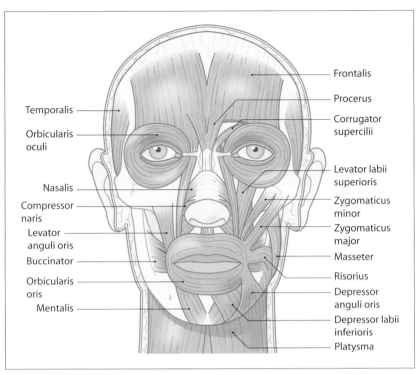

Frontalis

Procerus

Corrugator supercilii

Temporalis

Orbicularis oculi

Levator labii superioris

Nasalis

Zygomaticus minor

Compressor naris

Zygomaticus major

Levator anguli oris

Masseter

Buccinator

Risorius

Orbicularis oris

Depressor anguli oris

Mentalis

Depressor labii inferioris

Platysma

Fig. 10.1 Anatomy of the perioral area. (From Zide, B. M., & Jelks, G. W. (1985). *Surgical anatomy of the orbit*. New York: Raven Press Books, Ltd. With permission of Barry M Zide.)

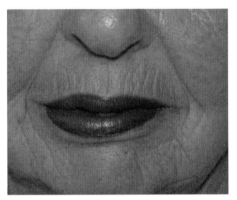

Fig. 10.2 Mouth droop following botulinum toxin for severe blepharospasm.

Treatment

Botulinum toxin causes a flaccid paralysis of muscles that have been injected and so induces a mild elongation as the muscle spindles stop contracting. This is particularly obvious in the vertical muscles of the face, for example in the upper lip. Almost all patients may successfully have their upper lip rhytids replaced with fresh smooth skin using CO_2 resurfacing, at different intensities and depths. Examine the patient carefully and consider the likely effect of elongating

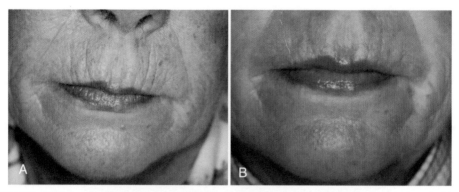

Fig. 10.3   **(A)** Before and **(B)** 1 week after first CO_2 laser treatment to shorten upper lip and soften deep rhytids.

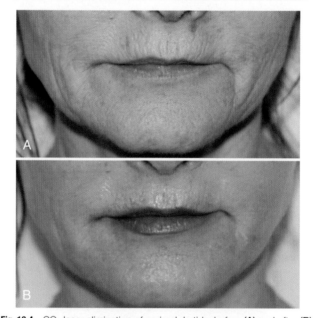

Fig. 10.4 CO_2 laser elimination of perioral rhytids, before **(A)** and after **(B)**.

a perioral muscle before injecting it. If the patient already has a long nasal-vermilion distance, for example (Fig. 10.3A and B), then treating upper lip wrinkles with further relaxation of the muscle will not produce a good appearance. Treatment of the nasolabial fold will also lengthen the upper lip. These patients can be offered alternative treatments such as surgery, CO_2 resurfacing and fillers (Fig. 10.4A and B) (see Chapter 11).

Perioral Indications

Upper lip rhytids
Lower lip rhytids
Pebbly chin
Elevation of lip corner
Reduction of nasolabial folds

UPPER LIP RHYTIDS

The author tries to avoid use of botulinum toxin to the upper lip unless absolutely essential. Some patients have small convex maxillae and are more prone to excessive resting tone of their orbicularis oris in the upper lip. Moderate rhytids, particularly in nonsmokers, can sometimes be discouraged with a small volume of botulinum toxin injected away from the vermilion border (Fig. 10.5). Limiting the contraction of the orbicularis oris will always curtail its true function as a sphincter around the mouth for articulation and eating. Patients often notice a weakening of their ability to 'pout' and, even though they seldom actually slur their speech, they sometimes experience the sensation of slurring.

More profound side effects occasionally occur, and patients must be warned about these. Milder sensations of poor articulation often wear off over the first few weeks. It is often easiest to counteract the risks by using a milder phased treatment augmented with resurfacing or fillers.

Whenever possible, encourage CO_2 resurfacing of the rhytids for at least a 50% long-term improvement (Chapter 11), or, if an instant remedy is desired, inject hyaluronic acid into the valley of the rhytid. Some patients benefit from both; but the author never recommends both at the same time in the lip or nasolabial fold area, to avoid inadvertent oedematous diffusion of the botulinum toxin.

If necessary, no more than 0.0125 mL of botulinum toxin per site (at the above dilutions) is recommended, subcutaneously. Using a lower volume at a higher concentration is also valuable, but difficult to manipulate at first and is perhaps best tried by an experienced operator.

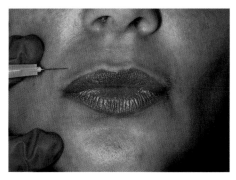

Fig. 10.5   Botulinum toxin (0.02 mL) to a superolateral rhytid in upper lip.

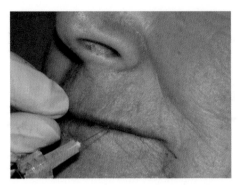

Fig. 10.6   Filler to vermilion border to treat 'bleeder lines'.

VERMILION BORDER

Fine 'bleeder' lines at the vermillion border can be injected with 0.0125 mL of botulinum toxin (Fig. 10.6). Avoid injecting rhytids farther away from the vermillion border at the same time. This minimises the laxity of the lip and the risk of side effects. Injections can be intramuscular or subcutaneous, depending on the patient.

Corner of Mouth

Botulinum toxin to the depressor of the angle of the mouth, just above the lower border of the face, 1 cm lateral to the angle of the mouth, can achieve a sought-after upturn of the outer corners, which can be nicely augmented with hyaluronic acid (Fig. 10.7). The depressor anguli oris is intimately associated with the underlying platysma and the adjacent depressor labii inferioris. Unwanted diffusion to the depressor labii inferioris will result in an inability to purse the lower lip, asymmetry when smiling, and even dribbling when drinking. Some experts recommend avoiding these side effects by injecting subcutaneously and not within 1 cm of the angle. Hyaluronic acid inferolateral to the lateral oral commissures, sometimes with some inside the lower and upper lip bordering the commissure, can often give a superior result to botulinum toxin here.

USER TIP

For perioral treatment, if in doubt, start with a low dose and low dilution of botulinum toxin, given subcutaneously. Review the patient within 2 weeks and give more if necessary.

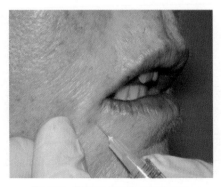

Fig. 10.7   Filler to lateral commissure.

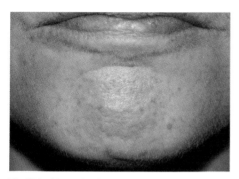

Fig. 10.8 Example of a pebbly chin before botulinum toxin treatment.

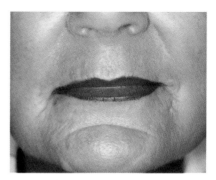

Fig. 10.9 Melomental fold.

NASOLABIAL FOLDS

Injections of botulinum toxin have been used to treat deep nasolabial folds, but the loss of tone in the midface is better managed with volume replacement. The larger particle size, for example Perlane, works well here, especially if initially layered on the superolateral aspects of the face (lateral zygoma, temporal fossae), creating a restorative 'lift', reducing the nasolabial folds and avoiding unnatural anterior facial volume changes (Chapter 11).

PEBBLY CHIN AND MENTAL CREASE

Botulinum toxin is excellent for smoothing the mentalis muscle, the main muscle responsible for wrinkling of the chin (Fig. 10.8). It is important to warn patients that the result may be asymmetrical at first, as the toxin may diffuse more towards one head of the muscle. Start with a low dose (0.025 mL) and increase this until the desired effect is achieved. Insert the needle directly below the centre of the tip of the chin, withdraw slightly having reached the periosteum, and inject 0.025 mL initially. Consider subsequent subcutaneous injections of 0.0125 mL to the overlying depressor anguli oris.

The mental crease deepens with age as the tip of the chin elevates (a 'Wicked Witch' chin). Hyaluronic acid (especially Perlane) will fill it instantly (Fig. 10.9).

Botulinum Toxin to the Neck

Botulinum toxin is very effective at neutralising the pull of the platysma muscle under the chin and so preventing horizontal banding lower down on the neck (Fig. 10.10). The author gives it to most patients with facial palsy to minimise the unilateral platysma band they usually develop (Fig. 10.11A and B). It is also effective in the treatment of 'turkey neck'—the vertical folds of platysma lying between the mandible and the clavicle. It is particularly good in combination with ultrasound, radiofrequency and CO_2 collagen stimulation treatments of the region.

The platysma spreads out from its origin at the base of the mandible and parotid fascia, down the neck and along the pectoral fascia. A reduction in the pull of the platysma tends to give the illusion of elevating the lower facial muscles and, in some patients, even of a reduction in their marionette folds. Treatment to the jowls (0.05 mL) and platysma bands sharpens the jawline and is known as the 'Nefertiti' lift.

Care must be taken to prevent diffusion of the toxin towards the oesophagus, which is extremely sensitive to it, as there have been several reports of unexpected dysphagia from earlier

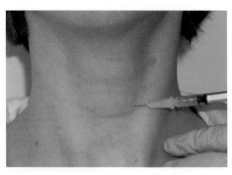

Fig. 10.10 Treatment of horizontal neck banding with 0.05 mL per site. The skin must be held between the fingers whilst injecting to avoid diffusion to the larynx or oesophagus.

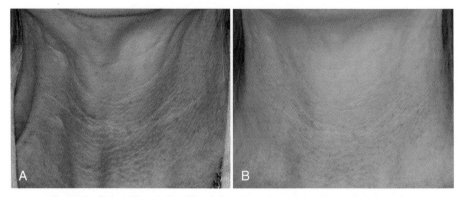

Fig. 10.11 Before **(A)** and after **(B)** botulinum toxin to neck in patient with facial palsy.

treatments, using doses similar to the frontalis ones. Care must also be taken to avoid the larynx as hoarseness has also been reported, along with difficulty in lifting the head. Divide the prominent area visually into units, and aim to space the injections of 0.05 mL 1.5 cm apart. Treat only the 'band' that is obvious at rest sitting upright, and not the flat part of the platysma that protrudes on effort. Treatment of the band often suffices and reduces the volume of botulinum toxin required (Fig. 10.12).

Finally, remember that some patients with prominent neck banding and 'jowls' would benefit from a lower facelift. Always discuss this surgical option with them and then refer them to a plastic surgeon.

Botulinum Toxin for Scars

Patients who normally heal well in other parts of their face tend to heal badly if they have a linear scar perpendicular to the direction of pull of a facial muscle. Muscle pull stretches and thins scars, which often remain red. This is particularly true for the frontalis muscle. The muscle can also pucker and 'dip', particularly in the perioral region and when parallel to the muscle action.

The traditional way of correcting unsightly forehead scars has been to re-excise them, taping the incision firmly with Steri-Strips and then bandaging the forehead for up to 6 weeks in an effort to keep tension off the margins of the scar. Botulinum toxin will provide a tension-free zone for up to 14 weeks (sometimes longer in the frontalis area).

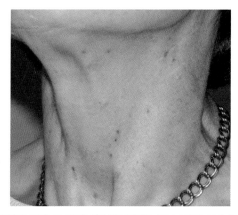

Fig. 10.12   Injection mark on neck of patient following vertical neck band treatment.

FRONTALIS SCARS

Inject the frontalis muscle evenly across the whole forehead, as in the treatment of rhytids (Fig. 10.13A) .This keeps tension off the scar while preventing asymmetry of the forehead, which would occur with injections localised to the scar itself. Make sure that every centimetre along the scar receives botulinum toxin, giving 0.5 cm on either side of the scar. The dose per site used is 0.05 mL.

PERIORAL SCARS

Great care must be taken to avoid the toxin diffusing towards the lip elevators or sphincter muscles of the mouth. Begin with the lowest dose, and increase this until an effect is achieved. Review the patient after 10 to 14 days to decide on this. Fig. 10.14A and B shows a scar that followed a road traffic accident in a patient who requested laser resurfacing. Examination showed that the scar was much

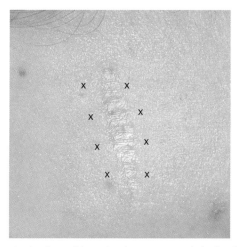

Fig. 10.13   Scar on forehead prior to excision, showing recommended sites for botulinum toxin before surgery. 0.05 mL at 'x'.

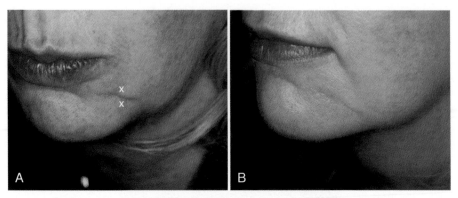

Fig. 10.14   Before **(A)** and after **(B)** botulinum toxin to scar on chin. '*x*' = 0.125 mL.

more unsightly 'in motion', that is while the patient was talking, than 'at rest'. BOTOX 0.0125 mL was therefore injected on either side of the scar, at sites 1 cm apart. The scar appeared to flatten over the next week and the patient was extremely happy. Follow-up treatment with the same dose, 14 weeks later, gave the patient the feeling of a 'drag' on that side of her mouth. This could not be detected on examination, but the botulinum treatment schedule was modified to annual sessions with occasional injections of hyaluronic acid as required (Chapter 11).

Décolleté

Multiple low concentrations of dilute subcutaneous injections in a 'v' shape to the décolleté reduce the sagging and accelerate remodelling with collagen-stimulating CO_2 resurfacing, radiofrequency and ultrasound treatments.

Other Solutions

Hyaluronic acid
Laser resurfacing
Upper and lower blepharoplasty
Combination treatments
Brow lift, neck lift, suborbicularis oculi fat lift
Fat transfer and nanofat injections
Collagen stimulating combination treatments
Dermaroller
Platelet rich plasma
Ultherapy ultrasound/radiofrequency
Skin protection and rejuvenation products

Introduction

Botulinum toxin is good at preventing wrinkles in certain age groups. It is the ideal treatment for 'wrinkles in motion' (dynamic lines) and can even dissolve 'wrinkles at rest' (static lines) in patients with good skin tone (see Fig. 8.2A and B). However, patients with poor skin tone, and deep crow's feet at rest, will not get a good response from botulinum toxin alone (Fig. 11.1A and B). Those with furrowed brows but a low lash-brow distance, poor tone of their forehead skin and/or an excess of upper lid skin (dermatochalasis) will actually look worse if they lose further muscle tone after botulinum toxin. They need an alternative treatment.

Ageing skin sags for several reasons. The skin loses collagen, becoming thinner and less transparent as the parallel collagen fibres become cross-linked and misaligned. This is greatly accelerated by smoking and exposure to ultraviolet (UV) A and B rays. The time at which ageing starts is genetically predetermined: if a mother does not have a wrinkle until the age of 55, then her

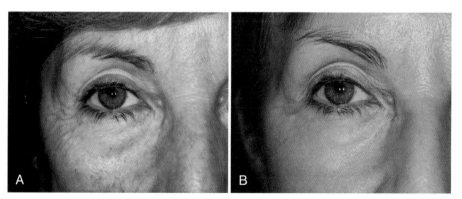

Fig. 11.1 Pre- **(A)** and post- **(B)** CO_2 resurfacing and botulinum toxin to static crow's feet rhytids.

daughter with the same genes and habits may not either. Clearly, the extent to which the skin ages also depends upon environmental factors. If a mother has had an excessive exposure to the sun and smokes, when she does begin to age at 55, she will probably become severely wrinkled within a short time. On the other hand, if her daughter—with the same genes—avoids UV damage and smoking, she may well retain the tone in her skin for much longer.

It is sensible to educate all botulinum toxin patients on the subject of skin protection and recovery ('stopping the clock'). Aesthetic nurse practitioners may spend time assessing the patients' skin regime and, if necessary, tretinoin (the author campaigns against cancer-causing paraben preservative in creams, etc.), paraben free, can be prescribed.

Ageing of the face is also due to the recession of its skeletal support. The anteroposterior diameter of the skull lessens with time, and this encourages sagging in spite of an otherwise excellent skin tone. The diameter of the orbit increases from superomedially to inferolaterally, reducing support for the orbicularis oculi muscles and skin. Traditional cosmetic surgery replaces this lost support by excising skin and muscle (facelift, blepharoplasty). Facial implants, such as malar and chin implants, have been used. The author favours the natural reinforcement of the foundations of the face with autologous fat transplant, using nanofat for the periocular tissues. Laser resurfacing can tighten and 'lift' sagging structures. Brow lifts are being replaced by brow repositioning (internal brow fixation or an endoscopic brow lift), while blepharoplasties often include lateral canthal tendon plication to tighten the sagging areas over an expanded orbital rim.

The tone of the skin is actively enhanced with collagen-stimulating treatments such as dermarolling and serum plasma injections. Autologous fat brings stem cells and plasma factors with it, further nourishing and rejuvenating ageing skin. Hyaluronic acid fillers are used to finesse periocular volume replacement, as well as supplementing lost skeletal support with larger molecule fillers such as Perlane.

The ways in which patients should be selected for botulinum toxin are discussed in detail in earlier chapters. Some alternatives (see Table 11.1) are discussed here.

Hyaluronic Acid and Other Fillers

'Fillers' are volume-replacing products that can be inserted with a cannula or injected into the skin. The principle behind their use is that, with age and sun damage, the face loses volume and so the skin sags.

TABLE 11.1 ■ Indications for Alternative Treatments with or Without Botulinum Toxin

Indication	Treatment
Crow's feet at rest	Laser resurfacing, platelet rich plasma, radiofrequency Viora Reaction, hyaluronic acid skin boosters
Lower lid bags	Laser blepharoplasty, fat transplant, nanofat remodelling
Vertical frown with low lash brow distance	Endoscopic brow lift, hyaluronic acid
Frown with heavy upper lid skin	Upper lid blepharoplasties, brow repositioning, hyaluronic acid
Upper lip rhytids, mouth zone rhytids	Laser resurfacing, PRP, Dermaroller, radiofrequency Viora Reaction, hyaluronic acid
Platysma bands, neck rhytids	Lower facelift, Threads, Viora radiofrequency, PRP, skin boosters, Dermaroller.
Poor skin tone, sun damage	Restylane skin boosters, PRP, Viora radiofrequency, Dermaroller. Microdermabrasion, chemical peels, tretinoin, alphahydroxy acid skin regime, vitamins C and E serum, sun protection

Fillers are an essential part of a good cosmetic botulinum toxin practice.

Fillers are an essential part of a botulinum toxin practice. Like botulinum toxin, they are injectable and associated with almost no downtime. Unlike botulinum toxin, the most advanced fillers give an instant result. Within minutes, a patient can leave the office looking up to 10 years younger. Many of our patients routinely book in for a 'top-up' of their filler at the same time as their follow-up botulinum appointment, to maintain their rejuvenation as the clock moves forward. Current legislation in Ireland prohibits the injection of botulinum toxin by a nurse practitioner, unless specifically prescribed by a doctor. This is allowed in other countries such as the U.K., and this handbook is designed to enhance a nurse practitioner's basic knowledge and safe practice with botulinum toxin. The same nurse practitioners are allowed to select and inject fillers and submucosal anaesthesia (but not nerve blocks). They are also experts in combination medical-grade collagen-stimulating treatments.

HYALURONIC ACID

Hyaluronic acid occurs naturally in the body and is the main component of the vitreous gel of the eye. It was originally derived from cockerel combs but is now produced synthetically. Since the 1980s it has been used extensively in cataract surgery to prevent the cornea collapsing and to protect the corneal endothelium during surgery. It is now available in different consistencies for intraocular injection. Restylane was developed by an ophthalmologist in QMed for injection into the skin (Fig. 11.2).

Hyaluronic acid is a pure substance, and the incidence of allergic reactions to it is very low. Patch testing is not required. Restylane and Perlane remain in the skin for nine months. Their molecules are gradually absorbed and replaced by water, which maintains the volume enhancement until the molecular framework collapses (Fig. 11.3).

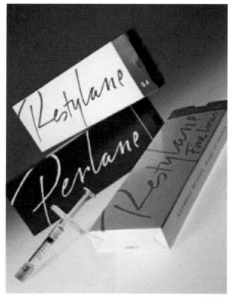

Fig. 11.2 Photo of Restylane and Perlane. (Courtesy Q-Med, AB, Uppsala, Sweden.)

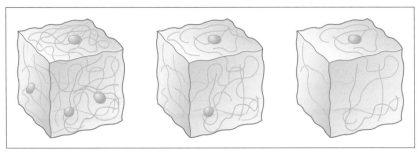

Fig. 11.3 Structural framework of Restylane and Perlane molecules. Initial volume is maintained throughout the degradation phase.

Many fillers are currently available on the market. Fat transplantation (the Sydney Coleman technique) offers a permanent solution, but is a semi-surgical procedure requiring time off work, and often more than one treatment session. At least 30% of the fat is absorbed, hence the need for a 'top up', but new microcentrifuged solutions of autologous fat (nanofat) are ideal for many oculo facial procedures, such as safe volume restoration at the superior and inferior orbital rims. A further benefit of autologous centrifuged fat is the accompanying platelet rich serum and its nutrients (the core part of a popular skin enhancing 'vampire facial').

In the past, routine cosmetic blepharoplasties included removal of all the orbital fat pads. The resulting gaunt look has long disappeared from fashion and volume is recognised as an essential part of youthful healthy skin. The author may sculpt fat in the lower lids, for example, but frequently transplants fat into the lacrimal fossae to restore rather than remove volume and minimise the dark circles under the eyes (Fig. 11.4A and B).

Hyaluronic acid is available in several ranges. The author continues to favour Perlane, Restylane and Restylane vital skin boosters by QMed. Skin boosters are popular for rejuvenation of face, neck, décolletage and hands, increasing hydration and elasticity for up to six months. Juvederm products appear to have a similar effect and the Belotero range of finer particled hyaluronic acid (Merz) is equally effective. Perlane, Restylane and Restylane fine line last for 9 months, but the author has evidence of Restylane fine line remaining in tear troughs for more than 24 months (Fig. 11.5).

The author's personal choice of product, based on experience, is currently as follows:

- Perlane appears to be the most viscous, most enduring and the best for deep rhytids.
- Restylane is of moderate viscosity, long lasting, good for deeper and superficial injections and the most versatile (d eep, superficial and lips).

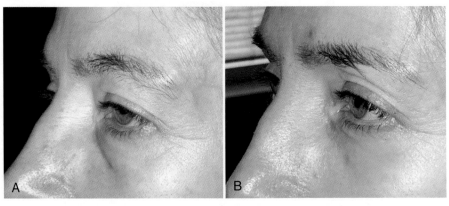

Fig. 11.4 Before **(A)** and after **(B)** autologous fat transplant to the tear trough.

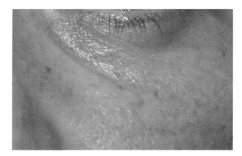

Fig. 11.5 Restylane filler remains in tear trough after 24 months.

- Restylane fine line and Belotero Soft come with a 32-gauge needle and smoothly fill fine superficial rhytids, for example crow's feet.
- Restylane skin boosters and Belotero Soft are ideal for nourishing skin.
- Sculptra (polylactic acid) is the synthetic filler of choice (if not using autologous fat) as a foundation in emaciated faces or faces with excessive lipoatrophy, for example after chemotherapy.

Indications

The choice of product depends on the area to be filled and on the volume required. Patients may also be restricted financially in their choice of treatment, which can be adapted to give the best value for their money. For example, Perlane may be best for deeper rhytids, but if a patient has both superficial and deep rhytids (e.g. a glabellar crease and nasolabial folds) and can only afford one syringe, 0.7 mL of Restylane may be used to treat both. Patients can be advised to plan for a full Perlane syringe in the future, and they should be made aware that the deepest rhytids compress the gel most quickly and require a top-up sooner. If there are no budgetary constraints, open as many syringes as are necessary to achieve the desired result (Fig. 11.6A and B). Failure to do so always leads to a dissatisfied patient.

It is important to analyse the facial features and then tell patients exactly what volume is required for an optimal result, for example 2× Perlane 0.7 for deep nasolabial folds; 1× Restylane classic 0.75 mL for lips; 1× Restylane fine line for cheeks. They will then appreciate that suboptimal results will be achieved with less and will not telephone the next day to say 'the lines are still there' if they buy only one syringe.

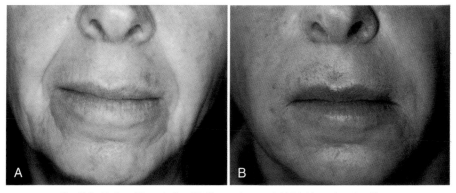

Fig. 11.6 Before **(A)** and after **(B)** filler to the nasolabial folds and perioral lines.

Patient Preparation

Injections of hyaluronic acid without local anaesthesia are sore—the pain being a sensation of pressure rather than the possible 'sting' of botulinum toxin. Injections are usually superficial and so can be effectively anaesthetised topically with proprietary lidocaine/prilocaine cream (EMLA) or lidocaine 4% cream (LMX). Deeper injections, for example to the lips, can be very painful. It is recommended to choose either a filler containing local anaesthetic or to infiltrate local anaesthetic submucosally first.

Patients should be warned that preparation takes at least 30 minutes. They should arrive early, in order that the nurse can apply EMLA and cover (with Opsite or Clingfilm) the area to be treated. They can then relax before treatment. For the lips, tetracaine gel is applied to the gums after these have been dried with a swab. A dental syringe with a short 30-gauge needle is used to infiltrate Citanest (or lidocaine [lignocaine]) submucosally in the fornix. This works in 10 to 20 minutes. Sterex antiseptic cream is applied after the treatment and the patient is allowed to apply make-up.

Nasolabial Folds

Some deep nasolabial folds are associated with a short upper lip and respond well to botulinum toxin treatment to the apex. Most deep folds, however, are best treated with volume replacement to the superolateral support structures of the face, replacing lost 'suspension' of the midface and therefore 'lifting' the nasolabial folds. Some patients require a surgical facelift, although it is not uncommon for a deepening of the nasal end of the fold to persist after an effective operation. Most patients presenting for botulinum toxin are not ready to consider major surgery at the time of their initial consultation and are thrilled to have a short-term 'cheat' with Perlane. Some will benefit from thread lifting, albeit for about 18 months before the threads dissolve.

Superficial filling can be very effective (Fig. 11.7A and B) and achieved either with Perlane or Restylane. Deep filling may take more than one session (Fig. 11.8A and B). Perlane may be placed in the superficial dermis of the nasolabial skin, deep to the epithelium. Deeper placement often fails to 'lift' the skin and may be 'lost' towards the sinuses. Warn the patient that this layer will become slightly compressed by facial movements and recommend a top-up over the same layer after 6 weeks. This compensates for the compression of the initial layer and achieves a long-lasting effect.

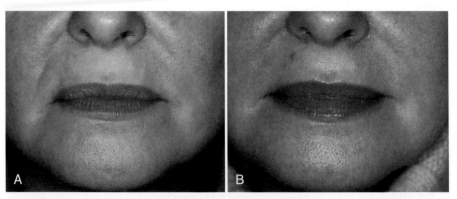

Fig. 11.7 Before **(A)** and after **(B)** treatment of fine nasolabial line with 0.4 mL Restylane.

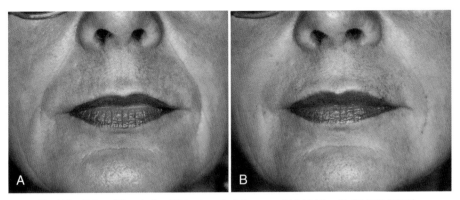

Fig. 11.8 Before **(A)** and after **(B)** treatment of deep nasolabial folds with Perlane 0.7 mL.

Marionette Lines

These can be improved greatly by lower facelift surgery. Some patients tend to slide their lower jaw back, emphasising the downturn of the corners of the mouth. Discuss the need for a dental opinion with such patients and refer them back to their own dentist if appropriate. The treatment of marionette lines with a filler is rewarding. As with the resolution of a frown, the elimination of these descending lines can alter a patient's countenance and create the illusion of lifting the whole face.

> **USER TIP**
>
> Do not overfill an area of skin with hyaluronic acid as this can cause local necrosis and bruising. It is better to bring the patient back after 6 weeks for further treatment to the same area. This allows for some compression of the initial gel and achieves a greater 'lift'.

Glabellar Crease

The treatment of a glabellar crease with botulinum toxin is discussed in detail in Chapter 9. Hyaluronic acid offers an instant 'fix' if a patient is waiting for procerus and corrugator muscle bulk to diminish. It is also ideal for those who are unsuited to full-blown botulinum treatment because of brow ptosis. The author favours Restylane for this area but has often placed some Perlane in the deeper dermis, or Belotero Soft or Restylane vital (skin boosters) more superficially. Usually less than 0.2 mL of hyaluronic acid is needed to treat this area. A small syringe (e.g. 0.4 mL) can be opened and sometimes the remains can usefully be placed periorally or nasolabially.

The Upper Lip

Patients complain of upper lip rhytids (especially smokers), or of a thinning of the upper lip, or both. The nose-lip distance elongates with age and some plastic surgeons shorten this surgically with an elliptical excision of skin from under the nose. Most patients are unaware of this elongation.

Overfilling of this fashionable area is not recommended as it increases the length of the upper lip, an ageing as opposed to a rejuvenating result. Deep CO_2 resurfacing of the upper lid not only erases rhytids, but also tightens and shortens the lip and is the author's treatment of first choice.

Look carefully before the anaesthetic is applied or injected. Ask the patient to pout and observe the gaps between the fibres of the orbicularis oris. Examine the distance from lip to nose.

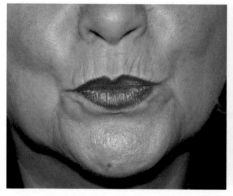

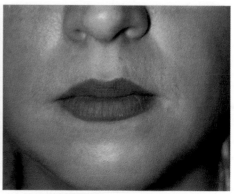

Fig. 11.9   Wrinkled upper lip emphasised by pouting.   **Fig. 11.10**   Cupid's bow/philtrum.

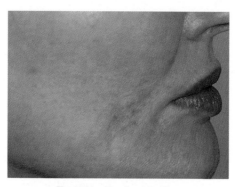

Fig. 11.11   Fine line injection.

Look for rhytids at rest and deeper rhytids in motion. Examine the symmetry of the lips and discuss this with the patient.

Care must be taken with 'wrinkles in motion only': inject Restylane into the gap that is seen with pouting (Fig. 11.9). Inject the superficial dermis and take care not to leave a bleb above the surface of the skin at rest. If a 'lump' forms, massage the area between two fingers and disperse the gel. Instruct the patient to do the same over the following few days.

'Wrinkles at rest' are always best treated with a combination of laser resurfacing and Restylane. Many patients will go ahead with fillers while waiting for the right time for resurfacing.

Restoring the convexity of the upper lip with injections between the orbicularis oris fibres shortens the lip nicely and improves its appearance. The philtrum can be reconstructed, again rejuvenating the lip instantly (Fig. 11.10), and often place a small amount at the Cupid's bow too.

Deep 'rhytids at rest' can be kept at bay with Restylane injected very superficially into the epithelium (Fig. 11.11).

Lip enhancement depends largely on taste. The author prefers not to enhance an upper lip that will protrude noticeably above the lower one, even if the upper lip is much thinner. It is not always possible to guarantee vertical volume, and in particular, with certain types of dentition, the gel can expand the lip anteriorly (Fig. 11.12A and B). Restylane is excellent for providing symmetry to lips. It is also useful for patients with cleft lip deformities, and when layered with Perlane, a nice anterior displacement of the upper lip can be achieved.

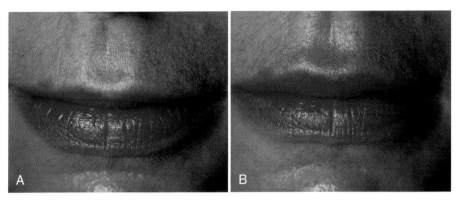

Fig. 11.12 Before **(A)** and after **(B)** Restylane to the vermillion border of the upper lip.

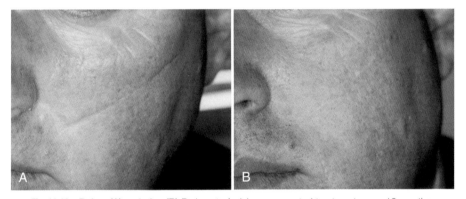

Fig. 11.13 Before **(A)** and after **(B)** Perlane to facial scar, repeated treatments over 12 months.

Scars

Hyaluronic acid is useful for the volume expansion of scars (Fig. 11.13A and B). Treatment with botulinum toxin is dealt with in detail in Chapter 10.

Crow's Feet

Botulinum toxin will erase some crow's feet and laser resurfacing will erase the rest (Fig. 11.14A and B). It is important, however, to identify 'hooding' before treatment. Patients with a fold of skin at the outer corner of their eyes will be disappointed with botulinum toxin if it is not demonstrated to them that their fold is due not to contraction of the orbicularis oculi, but to sagging of their lateral brows and temporal areas. In this case, the correct 'hidden-scar' treatment is by an endoscopic brow lift (Fig. 9.16A and B). Nanofat autologous transplant to the forehead reverses apparent volume loss with subtle restoration of brow positioning. Temporary correction of hooding may be possible by upper blepharoplasty. Some patients do not mind a lateral extension of their upper blepharoplasty incision, simulating a 'wrinkle', with extension of the scar along the crease, or sometimes with internal brow fixation (Fig. 11.15A and B). Patients are always advised that their hooding is obscuring their lateral vision and that surgery will rejuvenate, but also restore their lateral visual field.

Patients with hooding can sometimes cheat with Restylane fine line or Belotero Soft injected to the deep crease. The 32-gauge needle is inserted just below the epithelium, and gel is injected

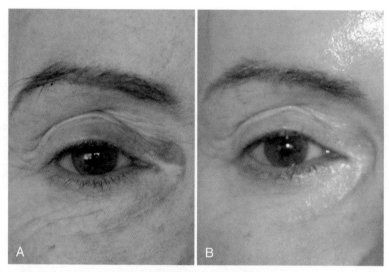

Fig. 11.14 Before **(A)** and after **(B)** eye zone CO_2 laser blepharoplasty (no surgery).

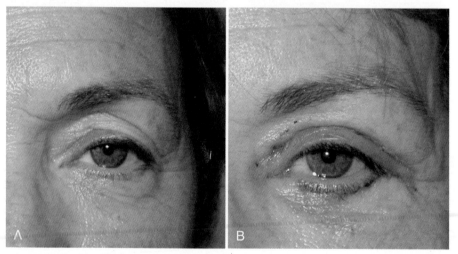

Fig. 11.15 **(A)** Pre- and **(B)** 1 week post-upper lid blepharoplasty with repositioning of the anterior levator muscle and extension of upper lid scar laterally to compensate for hooding.

along the rhytid. Another method is to place a series of gel micro-blebs. The result is an instant improvement, although some patients experience temporary oedema at the injection site. Fine line gel is also good for infraorbital rhytids, although laser resurfacing may be preferred rather than risk irregularities in the fine periocular skin.

The Chin

The use of botulinum toxin is an effective way of reducing 'pebbly chin' (Fig. 10.8). Perlane or Restylane may be recommended for irregularities in this area, particularly over dimples.

Cheeks

Botulinum toxin is not indicated for sagging cheeks: the treatment of choice is a mid-facelift or full facelift. Laser resurfacing will also tighten the cheeks significantly, but lost volume must be replenished with volume. An emaciated face, with or without lipoatrophy, will often benefit from a foundation of Sculptra. Autologous fat is a very good permanent foundation if the patient is suitable, with hyaluronic acid to the more superficial areas. The author has had considerable success with Restylane fine line to the fine rhytids of the cheeks, particularly those lying lateral to the orbicularis oris.

The tear trough may be carefully filled with Belotero soft, aiming to layer it deep to the orbicularis muscle to minimise the Tyndall effect. Fat injections work very well here, although they are less predictable (Fig. 11.5).

USER TIP

Avoid placing hyaluronic acid in the epithelium of a nasolabial rhytid, tear trough or the cheeks if the skin is fine and translucent. Translucent skin will show a blue grey mark of gel at the injection site (Tyndall effect).

Laser Resurfacing

Botulinum toxin is excellent for 'crow's feet in motion' and may diminish some 'rhytids at rest' with time. However, the complete removal of crow's feet is best achieved with laser resurfacing. Laser resurfacing is the treatment of choice for perioral rhytids, with or without fillers.

All of the results shown in this book were achieved with the Feathertouch (Sharplan) and Active FX (Lumenis) lasers.

Patient selection is discussed in detail in Chapter 5, but make sure that the patient is informed about static wrinkles and laser resurfacing before giving botulinum toxin. Failure to do so will lead to unrealistic expectations and disappointment.

USER TIP

Botulinum toxin is essential for the long-term results of the laser resurfacing of crow's feet. Counsel patients carefully about the natural return of rhytids after the laser resurfacing of crow's feet without paralysis of the orbicularis oculi (Fig. 11.16A–C). Suggest botulinum toxin injections are given a week before, and 3 months after treatment, as part of the resurfacing procedure.

Most patients who require botulinum toxin for crow's feet are happy to have the injections once they understand that their 'wrinkles at rest' may diminish and that the 'wrinkles in motion' will improve greatly. Most do not want the downtime of deep laser resurfacing, but can easily choose 5 days down time for superficial eye zone lines. It is important at the initial consultation to offer resurfacing as a long-term solution. If your practice is not involved in resurfacing, it is important to provide the following information—and a referral, if requested, to a laser practice.

Basic facts about laser resurfacing for wrinkles
- A laser vaporises the superficial layer of the skin, carrying the wrinkled layer with it.
- Treatment is under local anaesthetic for the eye zone and full conscious sedation for the face and neck. Eye zone CO_2 takes 15 minutes for crow's feet.
- The skin will heal in 5 to 10 days, depending on depth treated.

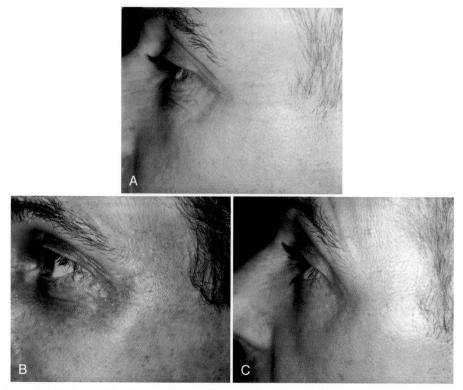

Fig. 11.16 **(A)** Before CO_2 skin resurfacing; **(B)** 6 weeks after CO_2 resurfacing: note return of crow's feet, before Botox; and **(C)** 6 weeks after Botox and 12 weeks after initial resurfacing: note wrinkles have disappeared.

- The skin will have ointment on it.
- Following treatment, the skin will be red, brown or even paler than the before.
- Freckles will be obliterated, providing a contrast with unfreckled skin. Intense pulsed light (IPL) may help blend.
- Treatment itself is painless, but simple analgesics may be needed over the first 24 hours.
- The patient must rest in an elevated position and apply cold packs for the first 24 hours to minimise oedema.
- The patient must be available for post-treatment examinations by the practice nurse—daily if necessary (rare)—for 5 to 10 days.
- The patient should take 1 week off work and socialising, although some can return to work with camouflage make-up after 5 days.
- The initial results will be greatly improved after 3 months when new collagen has been formed in the skin.
- Botulinum toxin is essential to keep the skin flat until this happens.
- The patient must avoid sunburning the new skin while it is healing.
- The patient must appreciate that sun exposure at 6 weeks will darken the treated area (postinflammatory hyperpigmentation). The use of a sun block is very important even though the pigmentation is reversible.
- Complete eradication of rhytids is not uncommon, but the patient should be warned to expect 20% to 50% improvement of the deeper ones.

- The older patient will still benefit from fat and/or hyaluronic acid injections for volume replacement as the 'new collagen' is often not enough.
- Non-lasered skin can be blended with the treated area by using IPL, Retin A, alphahydroxyacids, Dermaroller, chemical peels and sun block.

Upper Lid Blepharoplasty

Ageing patients who have an excess of skin over their upper lids (dermatochalasis) will often elevate their brows subconsciously using the frontalis muscle. This lifts the skin off their lids, restores the deep crease and takes 'the weight off their lids'. This excessive brow elevation will cause deep horizontal frown lines to develop. Such patients often ask for these wrinkles to be removed with botulinum toxin (as discussed in detail in Chapter 9). However, treatment of the frontalis with botulinum toxin will drop their brows to their lower natural resting position and accentuate the dermatochalasis. It is important to explain to these patients that they will look tired and older if their frown is paralysed. They must choose between frown lines and an upper blepharoplasty. Some patients may also need brow repositioning if their brows have sagged.

Some patients complain that using botulinum toxin for their forehead made their 'lids swell'. This is because a loss of brow elevation may also allow normal orbital fat to protrude. Figs 11.17A and B, 11.18A and B illustrate pre- and post-laser blepharoplasty patients. Making transcutaneous incisions and vaporising excess fat using a CO_2 laser reduces haemorrhage, oedema and recovery time.

If your practice does not perform oculoplastic surgery, then the following information may be given to patients, along with an appropriate referral.

Basic facts about upper lid blepharoplasty.
- Blepharoplasty means the excision of skin and/or fat from the upper eyelids.
- An incision will be made in the lid crease.
- The surgery takes place under local anaesthesia and lasts for between 30 and 60 minutes.
- Stitches will be removed between 4 and 7 days after the operation.
- The scar will usually be hidden in the crease.
- The patient must rest in an elevated position for the first 24 hours.
- Rest is important for the first 4 days to prevent late complications such as haemorrhage.

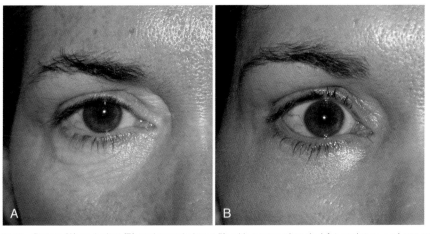

Fig. 11.17 Before (**A**) and after (**B**) endoscopic brow lift with transconjunctival fat sculpture and eye zone CO_2 resurfacing.

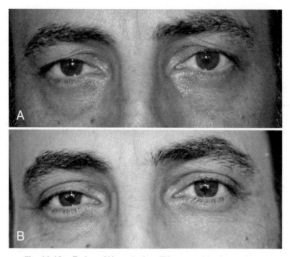

Fig. 11.18   Before **(A)** and after **(B)** upper blepharoplasty.

- One week off work usually suffices.
- The most common complication is bruising (reduced with laser incision).
- Rare complications include infection, prolonged swelling and haematoma formation.
- Results last until ageing causes further sagging of the skin, that is forever in some patients and at least 10 years in most.

Lower Lid Blepharoplasty

Ageing causes the skin under the eyes to sag. Laxity of the orbital septum behind the skin and muscle also allows the lower orbital fat pads to protrude, emphasising the 'bags', which are often held in the orbit by the tone of the orbicularis oculi muscle. It is very important not to inject botulinum toxin into the lower lid orbicularis muscle if it seems to be restraining fat in this way. Such patients must be told that they can only have their lateral rhytids (crow's feet) treated if they have lower lid blepharoplasties.

Traditional lower lid blepharoplasty is transcutaneous, through an incision underneath the eyelashes (subciliary). A skin/muscle flap is raised, the fat is excised, and the flap is trimmed and sutured (Fig. 11.19). Limitations to this procedure are a visible scar and increased problems with

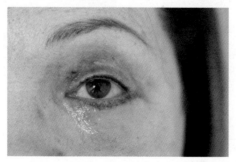

Fig. 11.19   Six days after infraciliary transcutaneous blepharoplasty (note blue continuous suture ready for removal), upper-medial fat pad vaporisation and eye zone CO_2 laser resurfacing (note ointment on post-lasered skin).

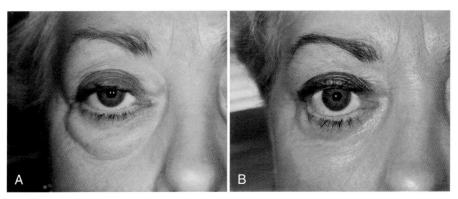

Fig. 11.20 Thyroid eye disease with protruding fat pad in patient with minimal infraorbital rim support and upper lid ptosis. Before **(A)** and after **(B)** upper lid ptosis correction and transconjunctival fat removal only to lower lids.

haemorrhage and bruising. It must be augmented with lateral canthal tendon reinforcement in patients with a strong negative vector, as with Graves ophthalmopathy, to avoid unattractive 'rounding' of the outer corner of the eye (Fig. 11.20A and B). Patients often combine transcutaneous surgery, if they have muscle sagging and require a trim, with CO_2 laser skin rejuvenation and transconjunctival fat vaporisation. (The fat may also be sculpted through the transcutaneous incision, but the author often favours retention of an intact orbital septum, particularly for patients with a strong negative vector who benefit from the extra support for their orbital fat.)

This procedure may be restricted to those who are not suitable for laser resurfacing, for example sun bathers with sun-damaged skin on their faces and no desire to blend old skin with new; patients with excessive orbicularis folds who require muscle shortening; and the many men who would find it embarrassing to wear make-up to hide the erythema that follows CO_2 laser resurfacing, which the author favours instead of excising excess skin (Fig. 11.21A and B).

> **USER TIP**
>
> Do not inject botulinum toxin into the lower eyelid if there is excess lower lid skin and fat. This causes the prolapse of fat, with protrusion of 'bags', until the orbicularis muscle tone returns.

The author prefers to perform transconjunctival fat removal. An incision is made through the conjunctiva in the lower lid fornix. Fat is then vaporised. This may be done without skin resurfacing (Fig. 11.22A and B), but most patients want their skin tightened too, and two passes with the CO_2 laser can achieve this. The type of skin can determine the choice of treatment. For example,

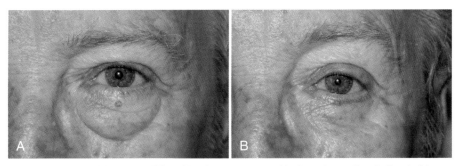

Fig. 11.21 Before **(A)** and after **(B)** traditional transcutaneous blepharoplasty with subciliary incision.

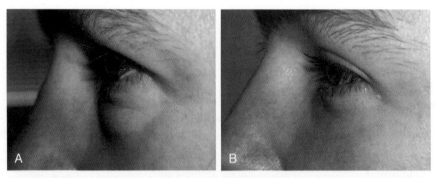

Fig. 11.22 Before **(A)** and after **(B)** transconjunctival fat removal with no CO_2 resurfacing.

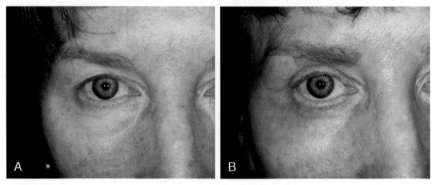

Fig. 11.23 Before **(A)** and 3 weeks after **(B)** deep CO_2 laser blepharoplasty with lower lid transconjunctival blepharoplasty and eye zone CO_2 laser resurfacing and botulinum toxin. Note pink discolouration that usually fades quickly.

Fig. 11.23B reveals persistent erythema, 3 weeks after CO_2 tightening of type 1 skin (extremely fair). This is easily camouflaged with make-up, but deep CO_2 laser tightening is contraindicated for someone who won't wear concealer. Such patients are advised to choose transcutaneous surgery instead of CO_2 laser. On the other hand, the patient in Fig. 11.24 had a more shallow CO_2 treatment (70 microns depth) with only 6 days of postoperative erythema and no long term sequelae, as seen 15 years later in Fig. 11.24C. Fig. 11.25A and B demonstrates four-lid CO_2 eye zone blepharoplasty with resurfacing, pre– and post–6 weeks with no make-up/concealer on skin.

Basic facts about lower lid blepharoplasty.
- This is the removal of lower lid fat bags with tightening of the skin.
- Skin can be tightened by excision with a cut under the eyelashes, or without a scar with a laser.
- If the skin is cut, the sutures will be removed between 4 and 6 days. There will be a fine scar, which can easily be concealed with an eyeliner pencil. Most people should take 1 week off work.
- If the skin is lasered, there will be no scar, but the resurfaced skin will take 6 to 10 days to heal. Postoperatively, the resurfaced skin may be red, brown and then pale (as above). Make-up can be applied as camouflage as soon as the skin has healed. Most people should take 2 weeks off work.
- The eye may be bloodshot after the surgery—due to bruising.
- The patient may require lateral canthal tendon plications (tightening of the outer corner of the lids through fine incisions in the upper and lower corners) to prevent 'rounding' of the eye contour.

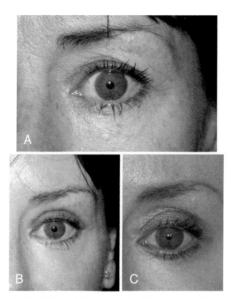

Fig. 11.24 Before **(A)**, 1 week after **(B)**, and 13 years after **(C)** upper and lower CO_2 blepharoplasties with superficial CO_2 skin resurfacing and botulinum toxin.

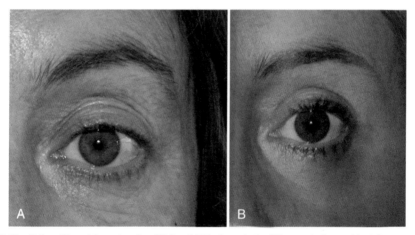

Fig. 11.25 Before **(A)** and 6 weeks after **(B)** four-lid blepharoplasty, CO_2 resurfacing and botulinum toxin in skin type 11, no concealer.

Combination Treatments

Some patients need botulinum toxin in combination with a filler, blepharoplasty and laser resurfacing to achieve the best result.

USER TIP

Do not give botulinum toxin injections at the same time as surgery. The effect may be altered by a local or general anaesthetic and in the author's experience has been unpredictable. In contrast, fillers, especially autologous fat, can be injected during surgery with good effect.

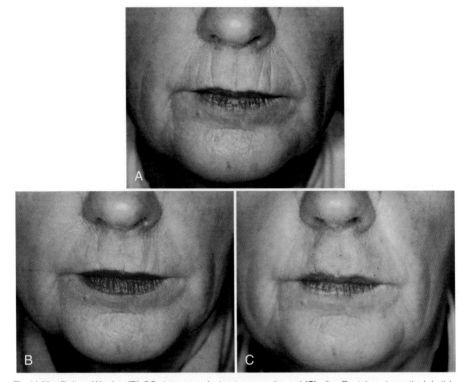

Fig. 11.26 Before **(A)** after **(B)** CO_2 laser resurfacing to upper lip and **(C)** after Restylane to vertical rhytids.

Lips

Fig. 11.26A shows a patient who underwent laser resurfacing of her upper lip. Fig. 11.26B is the same patient postoperatively, with residual clefts between her orbicularis oris rhytids. Botulinum toxin had little effect on reducing the depth of these. Fig. 11.26C demonstrates the lip immediately after an injection of Restylane.

Frown

Botulinum toxin will reduce the size of hypertrophic frown muscles—the 'mountains' on either side of the valley of the frown. The skin will, however, remain wrinkled at the point of chronic compression. Fig. 11.27A and B shows a patient who had Azzalure to her glabellar muscles, laser resurfacing of the sun-damaged rhytid and Restylane to the base of the rhytid.

Fig. 11.28A and B shows a patient before, and 3 months after, laser resurfacing and Botox to her glabella.

Face

Fig. 11.29A and B shows a patient before and after full-face CO_2 resurfacing including the upper lids, with Botox to crow's feet and frown and Restylane to upper lip and perioral rhytids.

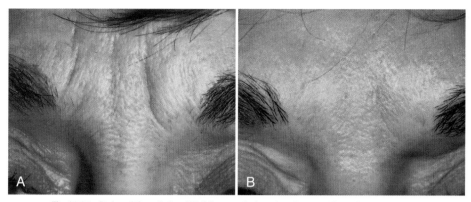

Fig. 11.27   Before **(A)** and after **(B)** CO_2 resurfacing, Azzalure and Restylane to glabella.

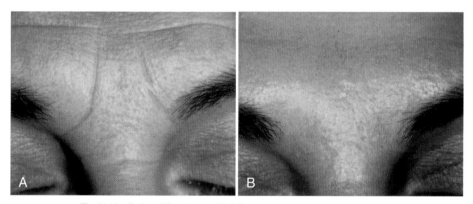

Fig. 11.28   Before **(A)** and after **(B)** CO_2 resurfacing and Botox to glabella.

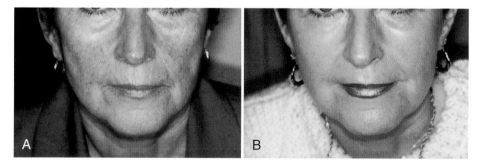

Fig. 11.29   Before **(A)** and after **(B)** full-face CO_2 resurfacing, Botox and filler.

Rejuvenation of the Skin

It is important when considering the management of crow's feet or frown lines to address the underlying causes. Inform patients that smokers have damaged 50% of the collagen in their skin at the age of 50 compared to non-smokers. Demonstrate their sun damage by comparing the skin on the inside of the upper arm with that on their face. Tell them that laser resurfacing might achieve the translucency of skin undamaged by the sun, but that this must then be blended in with the skin on their neck and the rest of their face.

An aesthetic nurse spends much time at the initial consultation explaining the effects of UVA and UVB on the skin, discussing different types of sun block and giving suitable samples. Interested patients can be provided with an anti-ageing regime that includes vitamins C and E and alpha-hydroxy acids. Paraben-free tretinoin 0.05% can be prescribed when appropriate. Such a regime, in combination with botulinum toxin alone, can provide dramatic results.

Patients who have booked laser resurfacing of their crow's feet with botulinum toxin are strongly recommended to have a course of IPL to the rest of their face.

Nonablative Collagen Stimulation

Patients are informed about nonablative collagen stimulation, for example, with Dermaroller, with IPL and with Viora radiofrequency to combat future effects of the ageing process. The author has developed pain-free solutions for all these treatments, allowing the patients to achieve superior results with little downtime and no pain.